D1532999

A Rendezvous *with* CLOUDS

A Rendezvous
with
CLOUDS

TIM FLEMING, MD

Foreword by David P. Sklar, MD
Afterword by Richard McCord

University of New Mexico Press
Albuquerque

Editors: Richard McCord and Ellen Kleiner
Cover and book design: Janice St. Marie
Interior photographs (in order): Lois Hirst, Jody Scioletti, David Hickey, and Barbara Deaux
Front and back (top) cover photographs: David Michael Kennedy
Back (bottom) cover photograph: David Hickey

UNM Press edition reissued 1999 by arrangement with Barbara Deaux. This edition contains the complete text of the first edition, published by Chamisa Press.

Library of Congress Cataloging-in-Publication Data
Fleming, Tim, 1945–1999
    A rendezvous with clouds / Tim Fleming ; foreword by David P. Sklar ; afterword by Richard McCord.
        p.   cm.
    Previously published: Santa Fe, N.M. : Chamisa Press, 1999.
    ISBN: 0-8263-2206-9 (pbk. : alk. paper)
    1. Fleming, Tim, 1945–1999. 2. Physicians—United States
Biography. 3. Indians of North America—Medicine—Southwest, New.
4. Indians of North America—Medical care—Southwest, New.
5. Emergency medicine—Southwest, New Anecdotes. 6. Cancer—
–Patients—United States Biography. I. Title.
R154.F676A3   2000
610' .92—dc21
[B]
                                                    99-37089
                                                        CIP

*This book is dedicated to Flynn Watahomigie,
elder of the Havasupai Indian Nation, who
taught me the important lessons;*

*And to my family: Barbara, Jesse, Adam, and
Chamisa—especially the children, who have
shared the gifts that only children can.*

With special appreciation to:

The talented photographers who have contributed their work
to this book: David Michael Kennedy, Lois Hirst, Jody Scioletti, and
David Hickey;

Three close friends who led me through the maze of
moving words to a finished book: Carl Hammerschlag, MD, Victor
LaCerva, MD, and Fitzhugh Mullan, MD;

My friend of twenty-seven years, Richard McCord, who
provided sensitive editing while maintaining my personal voice;

Ellen Kleiner of Blessingway Authors' Services, who gently
nurtured me through the self-publishing process, and
Janice St. Marie, who made the book beautiful;

As well as Ruth Kinsella and Mary Karshis, my adopted Irish relatives,
who reminded me of the songs.

Portions of these stories have previously been published in:
*The Santa Fe Reporter, The Pennsylvania Gazette, Bucknell World, JEMS
(Journal of Emergency Medical Services), Prehospital and Disaster Medicine,
Hippocrates,* and *Focus on Emergency Medical Services.*

Contents

PART THREE
GATHERING SHADOWS

Foreword

The first thing you would notice about Tim was his voice—whistling, cracking, and hoarse. He never explained or apologized for it, and after a while it just became a feature of his personal landscape like his thin angular face, his easy thin-lipped smile, and his attentive eyes. I am not sure when I found out about his cancer, probably about ten years ago as we discussed details of our lives at a dinner for emergency physicians. He was a survivor, he told me. I only connected the cancer with his voice when the cancer came back and he received radiotherapy changing his timbre, deepening it for a while, and then completely robbing him of his voice for a few days. Tim smiled and shrugged. "I've been living with this thing for a long time. I guess we have a few surprises left for each other," he whispered.

Tim became a member of my department four years ago, hoping to teach medical students and residents some of the lessons he learned from his patients and his own experience with illness. We often talked about writing down some of those stories, but he was busy with his duties as the State Medical Director for Emergency Medical Services, and it was only when the cancer returned that he embarked with a desperate fury upon the project that became this book. When he brought the book to me a few weeks before he died, I smiled gratefully. I knew it was his gift to all of us and I didn't care about its quality. It was enough that he had completed it before he died. I was almost afraid to read the stories for fear that they would detract from the peaceful, beautiful cover and his picture on the back.

But I did open it up. Some of the stories danced across the pages, others floated, and still others squeezed tears out of me.

His book is a precious gift of wisdom and compassion that speaks powerfully to healers and the sick, about the truths that Tim discovered as a doctor. I look forward to sharing it with residents, students, and professional colleagues, who are struggling with how to maintain their own humanity within an increasingly hostile medical care environment. And although Tim's voice is now silent, his words will continue to live on through these wonderful stories.

DAVID P. SKLAR, M.D.
April 1999

Part One

INDIAN WAYS

(June 1972–September 1982)

*I*n 1972, fresh out of medical school, I joined the US Public Health Service and was assigned to isolated medical clinics on the Hualapai and Havasupai Indian Reservation in Arizona. Every two weeks I would ride by horseback deep into the canyon to assist with their care. Within a matter of weeks I had developed the strong realization that this land and these people were home for me. My close relationship with Indian people continued for ten years and formed the essence of how I approached life's challenges over the next twenty-five years. Each step of the way it was evident that I'd gained far more from Indian people than I could ever have repaid them in healthcare services.

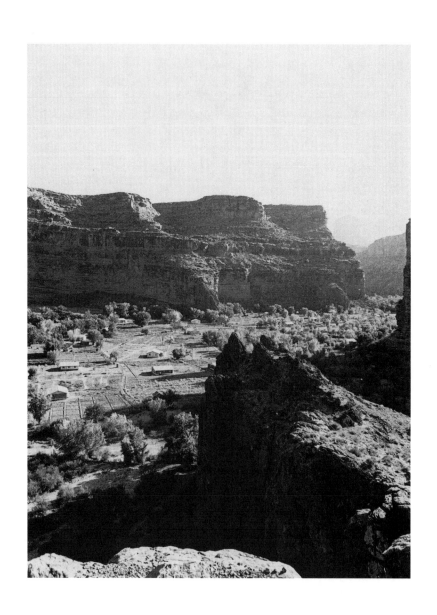

Supai

THE RELATIVELY NEW BUT WEATHERED JEEP rolls down the dirt road through the upper highlands of northern Arizona canyon land. The wheels grope for solid ground, but with the deep ridges, now hardened from the mud of summer thunderstorms, and the boulders jutting up from the earth, the vehicle is continually twisted and bumped and jostled on the route that is more a path than a road. The axles screech a coarse, metallic sound as they scrape rocks, and the motor whines as traction is suddenly lost, then gained again. It's not a leisurely trip, not one for sightseeing and daydreaming. The random, frequent lurchings keep the driver stiff and prepared for the flat tire or rock slide just around the next bend. Still, the sight of these broad plains interspersed with squat piñon pine and juniper are so overwhelming that a bit of daydreaming occurs nonetheless.

The sixty-mile journey through these Arizona highlands, rising 6,000 feet from the Mogollón Rim across the Kaibab Plateau, and onto the ridge of the Grand Canyon, is a journey of changing terrain. It begins with the seemingly endless rolling ridges of the plateau, sparse with vegetation. The road rises slightly as scrub pines dot the expanse. The evergreens gradually increase in size, in number, in configuration.

Suddenly, the road leads through a ponderosa pine forest—thick with foliage and color, mysterious, dark, almost foreboding. The road becomes less traveled, less rutted. The hands rest more steady on the wheel.

As rapidly as the pine forest appears, it vanishes and is replaced by flattened terrain and sagebrush carpeting the wide plains. The winding road sweeps ahead for miles like a ribbon. At last the daydreaming begins on this beautiful autumn morning, interrupted only by an occasional herd of antelope running and jumping across the horizon.

About fifty-five miles into the journey, when the steering wheel has become a dead weight from its menacing pull on my arms and the dust inside has built up to a point bordering on asphyxiation, my destination comes into view. There, four to five miles away, stands what could be the edge of the world. It is what most people know as the South Rim of the Grand Canyon. To the Indians who have lived in this land for centuries, it has another name: Hualapai Hilltop, overlooking an extension of Topocoba Canyon. It is the entrance to their ancestral homes around the Creek of Blue-Green Water. It is Havasupai.

The four-wheel drive finally struggles to a stop on what appears to be the most desolate parking lot in the world. Four or five other vehicles sit silently, deserted on a small piece of earth clinging to a sheer, 200-foot cliff of grayish sandstone rising toward the sky. No other souls are in sight. As I unwind from behind the steering wheel—thankful again that the road has been maneuvered—the only sound is a constant, whining wind rushing onto this precipice from 600 feet below. My workday is beginning.

As always—almost as if I must—I walk to the edge of Hilltop. From there the land falls perpendicularly 600 feet to a canyon floor and then meanders down a wash, falling still farther, where in the distance the red-and-white walls of the canyon formation rise higher and higher.

It's more than breathtaking. It's an important, almost religious experience and is the reason one feels small and humble in this land of the Havasupai. I silently look out over the canyons for many minutes.

The stillness of tall canyon walls and dry washes is suddenly broken by movement far down the canyon. At first subtle and apt to be mistaken for the wind blowing through brush clinging to the walls, the movement quickly becomes more obvious. Around a massive rock formation 600 feet below come one, then two . . . eventually five mules with empty packs. And finally, behind the distant figures, swinging his rope rhythmically, a single rider on horseback.

As if his presence opened a mystical gate, other signs of movement follow close behind. Another train of four mules rounds a rock formation far below. Then off in the distance, two men on horseback wind slowly up the wash to the base of the canyon wall. Minutes after the first sight, the sound reaches my windy perch. Hoofbeats— irregular and growing increasingly more intense—rapping and cracking on the rocks. It's a pleasing sound, countered by the faraway whistles and musical cries of the men as they push and coax their mules up the last, difficult stretch of that eight-mile journey from their village deep in the canyon.

My Hilltop solitude is replaced by a tempest of movement, sounds, animals and men. Earl Paya arrives first, then Hardy Jones, Floyd Putesoy, and Eljean Hanna. The mules and saddle horses, now tethered to metal posts on Hilltop, shake their heads to unseat the sweat from their journey and paw the ground to keep aging muscles loose.

Hardy demands news of Peach Springs, the village sixty miles away where I live and work, except for these monthly visits to the Havasupai. Peach Springs is the center of the Hualapai Indian Nation, a larger and closely related band of the Havasupai. Many families in the two villages are related, and the gossip is friendly, natural.

For the trip back into Supai, Eljean Hanna has brought from the village my horse—Ole Bill by name—a fourteen-year-old gelding going on twenty when he doesn't feel like making the journey for the trip into Supai. Bill, born and raised in Supai village, is powerful, individualistic, and cantankerous. I've learned he lets me ride only when the mood strikes him. He looks at me with those chestnut eyes, and we begin the process of psyching each other in preparation for the three hours we'll spend together alone on the trail. I give him a cookie to show good faith.

With the greetings and men's gossip completed, I throw onto Bill an old set of saddlebags that contain all the necessary supplies for three days in Supai: medical forms to be filled out, a few emergency drugs for the clinic, a stethoscope, an extra flannel shirt, a novel that never seems to get read, and a few cans of tuna fish for sustenance. Jumping up on Bill, I nod goodbyes and head for the top of the switchback trail.

Earl and Floyd will soon be packing their mules with the mail that comes by truck three days a week from Peach Springs. The mail is not simply letters, but food, supplies, furniture, anything that can be posted and placed on a mule's back for transport into the village. Hardy and Eljean will be packing down horse food, mattresses, and an old desk stored for weeks on Hilltop. Their day's work will end later in the afternoon, when the sun has gone behind the white wall and the village lies in shadows.

Alone on horseback this crisp fall morning, moving along the trail leading into Supai, I experience the recharge of energy that comes each month with the journey. The continual, unrelenting work in Peach Springs and the daily exposure there to poverty's effect on the human spirit have progressively taken their toll. By the end of a month—with no time off—I'm tired, frustrated, depressed. More importantly, I've lost the awareness that there is not just the agony of poverty in the present Indian existence but also a kind of joy that offsets every sorrow. That essential truth is always reaffirmed as I ride down the trail into Supai.

Swinging easily on Bill's broad back, I have a chance to stare at the formations along the trail and let my mind wander. Bill knows the trail well—he's made the journey thousands of times—and knows his next meal awaits in the village. Nothing short of a massive rock slide will deter him from taking the quickest route to that familiar place. He walks and trots gently while I stare at the walls.

A scientist by training, I know about wind and water on sandstone, and what millions of years can represent in terms of environmental effects. But the surrealistic formations that strike me at every glance transcend that knowledge. There is a sheer overhang here, a bas-relief on a large red rock there, and ahead high on the wall a shape that looks like a giant primeval bird. There is too much fun in fantasizing about huge animals and sculptured landscapes to wonder about eons of wind and water. It's nice to watch science become irrelevant.

The people of this land, the Havasupai as well as other Indians, believe that rocks have their own intrinsic, living spirit. They talk to rocks, and according to the people, the rocks answer if you listen well enough. That belief has typically been scorned by the white culture. But riding alone down the Supai trail, I sense the spirit of the rocks. Perhaps if I lived here and my ancestors had traveled these trails for centuries, the rocks would speak to me as well.

This mystical journey through the dry, stark canyons continues for two hours. Then coming through an especially narrow passage, I spy the familiar choir of tall cottonwood trees rustling in the morning wind. The smell suddenly changes, and living aromas fill my senses. The cottonwoods, many of them ancient, speak of a nurturing force, the reason this unique lateral canyon has been populated for centuries. For at their bases runs the ice-cold, crystal-clear blue-green waters of Havasupai Creek. It springs from deep grottos in the canyon floor three miles to the south and is fed by snow runoff from mountain peaks eighty miles away. It gives life to this otherwise barren canyon floor.

Ole Bill, smelling the creek's waters and sensing home nearby, begins an uncontrolled gallop that I'm unwilling to restrain. I share his excitement and we rush to the village about a mile down the canyon.

The village comes into view as we top a rise. To anyone visiting Supai for the first time, the village appears as a magical kingdom after the desolate canyons just traveled. The old wooden homes of the people are surrounded by newer, less functional prefabricated dwellings built through Bureau of Indian Affairs housing programs. Small plots of land are fenced off for the animals and for gardens of corn, squash, and melons. Everywhere there is activity—children playing outside the homes, women washing and hanging clothes, men repairing fences and shoeing mules.

Ole Bill strains at the bit as I hold him to a fast trot coming into the main village. He's eager to be home and unsaddled, but speeding is not tolerated here. The tribal police have been known to throw people in the single-room jail for such transgressions.

The Havasupai tribe numbers about 430 members. For thirteen centuries they lived a cyclic life based on seasons. Summers were spent on the fertile canyon floor, raising crops and escaping the heat through the cooling effects of the creek and forests of cottonwoods. In the winter, families would move south to the high plateau, where game and firewood were more plentiful. But as a result of presidential decrees and congressional acts beginning in the 1880s, the Havasupai were virtually confined to a 518-acre reservation in the canyon, as the south plateau became part of Grand Canyon National Park. In a seemingly improbable quest in the mid-1970s, the tribe successfully petitioned Washington to officially return ancestral plateau lands, and is now reclaiming ancient areas for winter use. Their lives, however, are a constant grope at survival under extremely harsh conditions.

"Hiya, Doc. How was the trip down?" Ted Schaeffer yells to me from behind his unshaven face and familiar Pall Mall hanging from his nicotine-stained lips. Ted is one of the few whites living in Supai, although his exact genealogy has always been open to question. Ted first came to Supai as a child accompanying his father, who worked with the Havasupai in the 1930s. He then left for more than twenty years to be a cowboy and landowner in Australia. But he returned many years ago, and has been here ever since, working for the tribe in a multitude of functions. His present job is helping with Supai Tourist Enterprises, the tribe's organization for controlling the influx of visitors who pour into the canyon most of the year to experience a magical string of hundred-foot falls on Havasu Creek as it works its way down to the Colorado River.

Walking with my saddlebags down the dusty main street to the clinic, I see familiar faces and exchange greetings. Although I am known in the village, I'm still a stranger to many, by their choosing. The people develop relationships with outsiders on a very cautious, reasonable basis. It is a trait I find most refreshing. Their culture and tradition demand it, for strangers can mean problems and bring change—often unwanted change.

I run into Carl Hillis along the way. "How you doin', man?" he asks. Carl has become a friend and colleague these past two months, for he has been living in Supai manning the clinic that serves the people. He is a well-educated, articulate Navajo Indian who has the official title of "community health medic," an Indian Health Service description of a physician's assistant. My visits to Supai once a month are primarily social occasions and a chance to check on patients with difficult medical problems; Carl handles the daily medical care for the people, accomplishing about 95 percent of what I am supposed to do. He is not only warm, sensitive, knowledgeable, and competent, but indispensable as well. And to the people of this village, he is their "doctor," their healer. Soon after arriving fresh out of training, he masterfully assisted in the delivery of a young woman's first child in the dead of night, then sang a traditional and ancient Navajo chant to the child, thereby ensuring the infant's strength and glory in this life. I admire and envy his powers.

The government clinic is a new, boxlike, prefabricated monstrosity that flies in the face of both aesthetics and functionality. Its only justification was its low cost and ease in construction from parts flown in by helicopter. The old clinic, used until a few months ago, was part of a weathered building next to the post office. That place had a personality. Even though our examination rooms were shared with spiders and other beasts of the earth, it was a place you could get involved with. The new structure, with its dull white walls and fluorescent lighting, leaves me feeling cold and uneasy.

Clara Hanna smiles shyly as I come through the door. She is sweeping the floor—again, for the dust generated by patients, visitors, dogs, and children who come every day needs constant attention. Clara has worked for the clinic many years and serves as receptionist, nursing aide, and housekeeper. We exchange routine greetings and news of Peach Springs, even though I've spoken to her countless times during the past four weeks on the sometimes operative phone line from Peach Springs to Supai. "How's our supply of medicines, Clara?"

I query. "I don't know," she responds immediately. I smile, for I admire her honesty.

With the cold winter months approaching and the troubled electrical system to the village sure to break down again, I consider the inevitable outbreaks of pneumonia and other respiratory diseases among the old and young. A quick check of the cabinets verifies my fears: the clinic is almost out of antibiotics and cough medicines. But we've got twenty-seven pounds of deep heat rub and three cases of milk of magnesia.

I pull out my order books and quickly scratch in what might be needed for the next few months. Such things are impossible to estimate with any accuracy. There are so many variables; if the people in the government warehouse in Parker, Arizona, are working, and if they have the supplies I need, and if the mails are functioning, and if the snows don't close the road to Hilltop, and if the switchback trail is not ice covered, then maybe we will have enough antibiotics in the village by winter to lessen the impact of illness on this small, isolated tribe.

I detect sounds from the waiting room. It must be my first patient of the afternoon. Walking in, I am greeted by the familiar face of a powerful elder of the village, Duke Idivica.

"*Gummo* . . . Old Duke," I yell, for Duke's hearing is not what it once was. This traditional Havasupai word of greeting is one of the few elements of their musical, guttural language I'm able to remember.

"*Hanneka*," he shouts back exuberantly. His smile and demeanor suggest he's doing all right and feeling well. He sits slowly in a chair, removes his worn cowboy hat, and wipes his forehead with his massive hand.

Duke's age interests me. His medical chart lists his birthday as sometime around 1880. He speaks of himself as being "'bout ninety years." Some village elders swear that Duke has been around the canyon for 100 years or more. It's an interesting but quite unimportant fact. Duke is simply an old, very wise man. His massive face is weathered like his hat, etched with lines of time. His pure white hair caps an expression that always appears ebullient. His vision is rapidly fading now, but a magnificent sparkle remains in his muddy eyes.

As regular as the rising sun over the canyon wall, each morning Duke walks the mile from his small shack down by the creek to the center of the village for a stop at the tribal store, the post office, the cafeteria (for coffee and stale pie), and the clinic. He comes in on the pretext of getting Clara to instill much-needed drops in each eye; but in fact, his visits are as social as they are medical. It's reassuring to be on Duke's list of important places to stop.

I sit beside him and once again attempt to absorb some of the history and tradition of this amazing person. He lived his days as a vibrant young man in a time when the whites were absent from the land of the Havasupai. His summers were spent in the canyon home, and his winters on the plateau. He longs to return to the plateau for a visit before he passes. We communicate in broken English, Havasupai, and hand signs about the weather, the children of Supai, and his remembrances of days past. I'm honored to be able to spend this brief time each month listening to him weave his tales of "the good day."

Then a steady influx of patients wanders through the clinic after trips to the general store for supplies. Many are people who come in each month for diabetes or hypertension treatments. A few patients with more acute problems arrive: an infant with pneumonia, a woman bitten by a dog, a young boy who has fallen and sustained a laceration. Between patients I attempt to repair the autoclave sterilizer that has not functioned in months, and rebuild a door frame. Before I know it, the afternoon has passed, the sun has fallen below the western white wall of the canyon, and the people are slowly making their way from the village to their homes along the creek. I sit quietly on the front porch watching the smoke rise from dinner fires and listening to the random barking of dogs echoing from the canyon.

The next day, morning and afternoon, I see more patients. Between clinic activities, I conduct physical exams on Head Start children and meet briefly with the Havasupai chairman to develop a joint tribal–Indian Health Service program that has recently become available.

Soon after lunch, Isa Uqualla urges me to make home visits to people who are unable or unwilling to come to the clinic. Isa has the official title of community health representative—a position that entails making home visits, performing liaison functions between the tribe and Indian Health Service, and developing new programs as needed. Powerful and well-respected, she has been a tribal council member for many years. She speaks softly yet persuasively on behalf of the Havasupai in their dealings with bureaucrats in Peach Springs, Phoenix, and Washington, DC.

With a few charts in hand and a kit containing the bare essentials of diagnostic equipment, we're off on foot along the dusty trails around the village. As we walk, Isa and I speak of political dealings, social situations, gossip, and her views of the future of her people. First stop: Mack Putesoy's.

Mack Putesoy lives about a mile from the main village, on the other side of Havasu Creek. His family compound of houses, round hogans, and corrals is massive. His sons have built a new prefabricated house, but Mack chooses instead to stay in the old wood-burning shack that has been his home for decades. Although suffering from a multitude of health problems, Mack gets around fairly well. In another environment he might be chronically hospitalized, but in Supai the best therapy is his daily excursion to the sweat bath that almost magically keeps his body and spirit strong enough to continue living. I have no further suggestions for old Mack, and feel powerless to help him. But in the visit alone there is something we both feel.

After walking another mile back along the creek, through an obstacle course created by barbed-wire fences outlining family land and corrals, Isa and I reach the small yet complex home of Kati Hamidreek. Kati, about sixty-five years old, recently had a bout of what might have been gall bladder disease. (Such diagnostic conclusions are at best a guess in this context.) She was in pain for days, but between my "modern" medicines and her traditional therapy of placing on her stomach warm rocks wrapped in burlap, Kati seems back to normal. She is squatting on the ground, her wide skirt forming a round base in the dust, cooking flour tortillas on an open fire.

"How you feeling, Kati?" I ask. She simply smiles and nods her head and continues to hand-roll the dough before her on the ground. With business out of the way, Isa and I sit on the earth with Kati, share news of relatives in Peach Springs, and join her by the fire for an afternoon meal of tortillas and warm beans.

Isa tells me our last visit should be to check on Elva Watahomigie, Clara's mother, who has not been feeling well the last few days. We find Elva inside her little house, wrapped in blankets on her old cot, not looking at all well. After gathering a bit of history and obtaining a sparse exam, I draw no definite conclusions, but empirically sense she has the flu, with complications stemming from her age and underlying diabetes. I leave a symptomatic treatment and make arrangements for Carl and Isa to check her in the morning. If she hasn't improved at all by then, I'll arrange for the costly helicopter and airplane evacuation from Supai to the Indian Medical Center in Phoenix. Feeling useless to do more, I slowly walk back to the clinic with Isa as the falling sun transforms the cottonwoods into a brilliant display of colors and shadows.

There are ten more patients waiting at the clinic. It's past five o'clock before I have a chance to relax with Isa over a cup of coffee in the clinic's small kitchen. But then, Clara peeks through the door and says, "One more patient for you to see out back."

"Out back?" I complain. The day has been long.

Walking to the rear of the clinic, I discover my last patient. Young Toby Watahomigie is standing there, holding on to a rope and harness attached to a massive, snorting two-year-old stallion. The horse has obviously run into barbed wire and is sporting a large, open gash on his shoulder. Something, of course, has to be done. And in Supai, the people and I make little distinction between medical and veterinary health care. I do the best I can with the stallion: clean the wound, apply antibiotic ointment, and give him a massive injection of a thick, white penicillin-streptomycin solution. In the process the horse almost tramples me to death, along with the four boys trying to hold him.

That night after dinner, Carl and I walk silently along an

unmarked trail that leads from the village up the side of the canyon's 200-foot red-wall formation. In the near darkness, the rocks are hazardous and I stumble frequently. Carl has less difficulty, for he has a sense about such things. We wind our way cautiously to a cliff that juts out over the village far below, where a few gentle lights from houses flicker magically. The stars overhead—bordered by the canyon walls—are cosmic in intensity and effect. We sit silently, not wanting to impose hollow words onto the solitude and beauty of this place. We sit silently for a very long time.

After an interlude in which all perception of time is lost, I notice that the 1,200-foot white-faced wall to the west has become more visible in the darkness. I watch this change with awe and confusion, for my senses haven't been altered this evening by any agents known to cause such things.

Soon the reason for my altered perceptions becomes obvious. The moon, massive and almost at fullness, rises over the eastern wall and illuminates the canyon with a light of immeasurable brilliance. The western white-faced cliff stands stark and tall with a luminescence that a theater spotlight might create. I sit in silence, filled with the vast insignificance of small problems that occurs when we let it. And a full, warm tranquillity comes with the darkness.

Tomorrow I'll ride out on Ole Bill at the first light of dawn. The long trip by vehicle back to Peach Springs will leave me weary but rejuvenated. For the moment, there is nothing in the universe save that white-faced facade illuminated by the moon, and the little village falling to rest for another night.

Sing the Songs Again, Old Duke

THE OLD MAN WAS AN INDIAN. He was called by many names, but answered most often to Duke. Old Duke Idivica. But Duke would answer only when his name was shouted loudly, for he had developed a problem with his hearing. It came with age.

His age was a point of constant contention around that small Indian village. Duke could be found leading the arguments as the old men sat in front of the general store watching the days go by and talking of things. They spoke frequently of the past—especially of when the white man was absent from their land, life was more reasonable, life was Indian. It was not that way anymore, so when the old men talked, they spoke most frequently of stories from the old days when things made more sense to them.

The men's arguments were usually about Duke's age, for he claimed to be the oldest man in the village. His record at the small medical clinic had his age as 95. Other documents put it as 98. Duke claimed that he was well over 100. Old Beluah Wescogame scoffed at that. Hell, he had known Duke as a young boy, and was sure he couldn't be that old. The debate continued almost daily, with no agreement reached but good talk passed in the process.

Everyone agreed on one thing: Duke was a very old man who had much to tell of both his days and the days of his people. When Duke began his stories, everyone listened for the breath from the past.

I remember seeing him there in front of that small general store, sitting on a bare wooden bench. Someone had thrown an old worn plank, too warped for use in construction, between two cinder blocks placed on end. An old warped board, but a fine bench for sitting and watching the children grow as the days passed on.

Before arriving at the bench, usually by late afternoon, Duke would make his daily rounds of the village. He would arise early with the morning light, at his hut about a mile away. He had lived alone there for fifteen years, ever since his last wife died. For the old man it was time to live alone. He didn't have enough energy left to be living with someone else.

Moving slowly, carefully around the dirt-floored hut, Duke would prepare a simple breakfast. His tired legs and stiff muscles would soon loosen, although it took more effort each day as the cold wisps of fall wind rushed into the canyon. Then with his dog by his side and his cane in hand, Duke would start the slow, steady walk into the village. The trail was dusty and irregular. Steps were taken slowly, carefully. There was no great hurry, and any foolish step could lead to a fall from which he might not rise. Vision played little part in his journey—his eyes had long since failed him and now let in only diffuse light and hazy patterns. His steps were guided by other means; he had walked that trail countless times, and could sense every rock, every irregularity.

Duke would hold his hand-carved cottonwood cane upright, ready to take a sharp but kindly swing at any dogs that rushed toward him and his companion. The dogs of the village knew Duke's cane well and respected its language.

By the time the sun was noon-high over the land, Duke would slowly wind his way into the main village. The people who passed him would call out, "*Gummo*, Old Duke—how you doin'?" A grin and a nod of the head would answer them all. Duke was fine and was coming into the village again.

His first stop would be the small cafeteria tucked into the community center. After working his way through the heavy doors, he would sometimes be jostled by small children rushing and playing about the room. He would look in their direction with benign gruffness and purse his lips, shaking his cane ever so lightly, as he did with the dogs. The children would giggle yet remember the lesson. They would be more careful next time.

He would make his way to the nearest chair his hands could find, take a seat, hang his cane over another chair, and stare off into the shadows that filled most of his visual world. Ester or Edith or whoever was behind the counter would see him enter and would smile warmly. Within minutes, she would bring to Duke's table his dark, hot coffee and a piece of pie or cake—whichever was available. Invariably, it would be stale, since getting fresh staples into that isolated village was difficult. But it didn't matter to Duke.

He would nod his head with thanks in the direction of the waitress and proceed to pour sugar into the thick white mug. For minutes, he would slowly stir the dark liquid with sweeping motions of his spoon, making high-pitched clinks as it struck the heavy ceramic edge. He would take small bites of the pie, slowly gumming its sweetness. Duke took his time with such things, as is the way with old men.

After the traditional pie and coffee, he would work his way across the village's dusty main street to the post office to visit Virginia Hanna, the postmistress. Rarely was there a letter for Duke—although sometimes he would receive a circular, or a notice from the government concerning some new program it had initiated, or a catalog from a mail-order house. Virginia would read to Duke from the mail. He would sit and listen quietly, paying attention to all her words.

Then he would begin another slow stroll up the main street to a small clinic at the end of that long row of cottonwoods. When Clara Hanna saw him walk carefully through the front door, she would go to her cabinet for the eyedrops he received daily. Duke would exchange brief greetings with others at the clinic, then sit in the waiting room's largest chair as Clara would instill the drops in each eye, causing him to wince from the sudden sting. Then he would rest quietly, head slightly back, eyes closed, hands folded across his lap, while the drops brought back a measure of moisture to his tired eyes. He would sit that way for a very, very long time as the life of the village went on around him.

Finally, after thanking Clara a second time and finding his way out the door, Duke would end his journey at the weathered bench in front of the store. There he would take his seat and wait for other villagers to gather in late afternoon before making their way back home for the evening meal.

I remember him sitting there every day. It was a pleasing and reassuring sight, like watching the sun strike the canyon wall each morning. His hands would rest on that old cane, holding it in front almost like a scepter. His head would move back and forth, tracking the shadows cast by horses and people as they moved by. His large black cowboy hat, stained with sweat and dust, covered his large head of short, dense white hair. His dark face was etched with lines of time and experience. His thick, black-rimmed glasses hid his eyes, but one could almost sense a sparkle remaining in the worn globes. His flannel shirt hung loosely from his body, and his faded jeans gathered more dust from the horses and people passing.

He was a pleasing sight there on that warped bench each afternoon.

There was a story told about Old Duke, from the previous summer. I wasn't in the village at the time, but the story was told by those who were. They remembered the day well and told the story often so that all would remember it. It happened late one afternoon.

Duke was sitting in front of his wood-and-mud hut, feeling the day go by. A few people had gathered there with him—the Hanna boys, Harjoe, and a few others. They were speaking, as usual, of the past and listening to stories of those days.

One of the boys asked Duke about the Rain Sing. Such songs were not sung anymore, but the boys knew that Duke was the last surviving member of the tribe's family of rainmakers. His clan was the one that knew the important chants and prayers for bringing rain to the parched earth. His family had passed the chants down from generation to generation. It had been the way for longer than anyone could imagine. Duke's father, Old Burro, was the best rainmaker that ever was. Anyhow, that's how the story went.

Duke's family not only had the words and prayers for bringing rain; they also had the Power. That was as important as the words. One had to have the Power to bring rain to the crops. It was through the Power that the sky would respond.

Old Duke sat silently for some time, thinking about the question. The boys watched him closely, knowing inherently that such answers come when it is time for them to be heard. They, too, sat silently.

Finally, Duke began to speak of the old days. He spoke of how the rains were needed for crops of corn and squash and melons. How the rains came rarely during those hot summer days. And how the rains came from Father Sky when the people sent up prayers for the crops. The crops meant life for the people, and it was only through their prayers that the rains would come. Such things were connected. Such things were part of the life.

He stopped talking and sat back, reflecting on things beyond words.

One of the boys asked Duke to sing them the songs. The boy wanted to hear the old sounds that brought rain to the earth.

Duke shook his head slightly. No . . . he couldn't remember how they went. It had been too long since he had sung to the sky.

The boys pressed on. "Just give us a sound," they said. "Just give us an idea of how it was."

Duke sat a while longer, his eyes closed tightly. Some of the boys thought they saw tears dripping down his cheeks, but they could not be sure.

Suddenly, the old man put back his head and began a low rhythmic chant in the old tongue. It was soft at first, barely audible, and seemed more like a moan than a song. Then his shoulders began moving back and forth, one foot tapped regularly on the dusty earth, and his cane moved up and down against the ground, in time with his voice. The voice grew louder, becoming more powerful, singing a song as old as the walls from which it echoed. It grew in intensity as Old Duke remembered the lessons of generations. He had not forgotten.

Duke went on singing the song for ten, perhaps fifteen minutes with the insistent chant now full-voiced and moving. The boys watched in awe. This time, tears on the cheeks of the old man were obvious—there was no longer any doubt.

Suddenly, he gasped for breath, seemed to choke for an instant, then stopped singing. The silence of the canyon walls and cottonwoods blowing in the afternoon breeze filled the void. Old Duke quivered and shook his head.

"I can sing no more today," he said. "The song is too powerful. It is not good to keep singing. I must stop this song."

Duke rose and walked into his hut without saying another word. The boys sat on the ground staring at his doorway, reflecting on what had just happened. After a while, they rose and began walking back to the village. They spoke briefly about the old man, but most of their time on the dusty trail was spent in silence.

Soon after they arrived in the main village, a rumble was heard off in the distance, beyond those canyon walls. The deep blue sky filled with gathering clouds, dark and powerful. Within an hour, the sun was gone, the heat had disappeared from the air, and a wind had come up strong and moist. Horses became nervous and snorted in the wind. Women ran to their clotheslines; men hurriedly threw canvas tarps over their saddles and packing gear.

Rain began to fall. At first, it came in big intermittent drops, but then the skies opened in a torrent. The sun hid for two days, most of which were filled with a steady, unrelenting rain—the kind the neighboring Navajos called a Female Rain. Steady, gentle, nourishing.

Duke was not seen for three days. He didn't come into the village for coffee and pie and eyedrops. Neighbors near his hut swore they didn't see him leave his dwelling all that time. After the clouds had gone and sun returned to clear, blue skies, Duke walked back into the village, as he had done countless times before. His demeanor seemed unchanged. It was just good old Duke coming into the village as always.

While eating his stale cake and drinking his sugary coffee at the cafeteria, he was joined by one of the Hanna boys, who remarked about the recent events that had occurred. Old Duke looked in the boy's direction and smiled his big toothless grin.

"Have to be more careful," he said. "Forgot how powerful those songs are . . ."

Returning to his cake and coffee, he finished them in silence. It was time to move on to the post office.

Supai Dogfight

THAT GENTLE SPRING AFTERNOON in the small Indian village of Supai was like most in that timeless place. The sheer 600-foot canyon walls on either side of the village stood tall and red. The canyon floor, verdant with new crops and cottonwood leaves, glowed in the bright sunlight. A deep and cloudless blue sky crowned the canyon walls. Gentle breezes from the south murmured musically in the budding cottonwoods.

Through the village rushed the blue-green waters of Havasu Creek, cold and clear from the winter's melting snows far to the southeast, in the mountains around Flagstaff. As the sun struck the crystal liquid, turquoise color exploded in rivulets of movement. Almost all the lateral passages along this stretch of the Grand Canyon are dry and desolate; but in Havasu Canyon the creek brings life to the thin soil, and greenness to a world of barren rock.

The people of the village were going about their afternoon tasks. The makeshift cafeteria and community center teemed with women and children seeking gossip and cold soda pop. On the dusty ground outside, children played the games they have always played in that quiet village. No store-bought toys were needed—a simple stick would do, or some rocks and a board. The games had no names, and no definite beginning or end. They filled the bright spring days.

The general store was busy with afternoon shoppers preparing for evening meals. Because few people had refrigerators, food was purchased on a daily basis. The store was another place for meeting friends, for passing the gossip. Women were leaving the store with their simple canvas pouches thrown over their shoulders, filled to capacity with beans, flour, sugar, bread, whatever small amount of stew meat might have been available.

Mounted men and boys moved along the dusty main street of the village. The boys rode sometimes two or three to a horse, their little bodies nestled into the curved back of an aging gelding. They raced down the corridor, unaware of or unconcerned about the infrequently enforced speed limit for horses. Occasionally, a very young child, just three or four years old, rode by, knees pressed tightly together, tiny hands on the old leather reins.

As the sun dropped, men on horseback filed quietly by the store, heading home from their long day on the rocky trail linking the village to Hilltop, an isolated precipice of canyon wall where supplies, mail, and staples of life came in by truck three times a week. The day had been long. The men had been up before dawn, before the first sun struck the west canyon wall. In the cool morning air, with saddle horses and pack mules tied together, they were well up the eight-mile trail. But after the packing and storytelling at Hilltop, they could not get back to the village before late afternoon. Now with their workday ending, their broad dark faces showed they were glad to be home. Calls and smiles greeted them from friends entering and leaving the store.

Out in front, on a weathered board between two cinder blocks, the older men held forth. There they sat, watching village life go by, telling stories of the past. They shared much good conversation, much laughter.

It was a good spring afternoon in that quiet village.

And then there were the dogs, hundreds of them, of all shapes and varieties. An exact count of the dog population was impossible. But with 430 tribal inhabitants of Supai and each family casually claiming two or three animals, plus another forty or so feral members of the pack, there were probably more dogs than humans in the village. Dogs with long coats and dogs with short, bristly coats. Dogs of solid brown and dirty white and off-yellow. Dogs with stubby noses. Dogs with floppy ears. Dogs that belonged to people and dogs that simply roamed, living off the refuse of the village. Dogs that were known to all. And dogs that never had a name.

The village's canine population was astounding. It multiplied, as dogs do, and any attempt at licensing or control was out of the question. It was a moving population with its own social order and hierarchy. Every two or three years, under the prodding of some federal official, the dogs were gathered and vaccinated against rabies. The most scruffy of them, if unclaimed, were destroyed. But one youngster or another usually claimed a loose connection with some mutt, hence few met the fate of a cold injection of barbiturates. So despite the obligatory roundups, the dogs remained an unrelenting sector of Havasupai society, one that rarely caused damage and coexisted in harmony with other living things in the canyon.

They gathered, as did the people, in late afternoon. Life went on around them, between them, over them. They played their own games and sunned themselves outside the cafeteria. Only when they inadvertently blocked the doors would someone send out a kick and yell the universal word of castigation: "*Sama!*" It was a powerful word—one that worked, as had been discovered, with dogs of all tribes. Even dogs belonging to white people understood it. It was a multidialectical pronouncement, especially when combined with a sharp kick or swipe with a stiff stick.

Despite occasional misunderstandings, quickly forgotten by both parties, the people and animals and cottonwoods of Supai usually just went placidly about their business. But every month or so, as if some grand timepiece ticked off the inevitable necessity, an event occurred to disrupt the tranquillity. Suddenly, inexplicably, and spontaneously, a Supai dogfight would erupt.

No one was ever sure what started the fights. Few people noticed or really cared. The combat zone would vary; there was no favorite battleground. The dogfights would simply happen when the time was right and a critical mass reached. There was no predicting the event.

Once, a grand and unforgettable fight exploded while a visiting party of dignitaries from an Eastern university was touring the village. Paralyzed by the event, the professorial visitors took the next available helicopter back to the canyon rim and the safety of civilization. Another time, a Supai dogfight lasted more than an hour, lowering the canine population so drastically that it stayed at a depressed level for more than two years, negating the need for public health officials to come by on their regular roundups.

And remarkably, in an event remembered by many, a fight began one evening in the middle of the small community center during a performance by a classical-music string quartet from Tucson. As with all events in the center—be it a tribal council meeting or elementary school Christmas play or rare concert by a visiting group—when the villagers gathered, with them came the dogs. Doors were rarely closed in village buildings, so it was commonplace to have fifty or so tribal members sitting on folding chairs with almost as many dogs resting lazily underfoot while the business of the evening was being conducted.

That particular evening, in the midst of a melodic Mozart divertimento, with most of the villagers in attendance falling asleep, some thirty Supai dogs began a violent quarrel, clearing the room of audience and musicians in seconds. Chairs went flying. The cellist and violinist ran for their lives, clutching their instruments in a frenzy to make it to a door, to outside, to safety. The concert never resumed, much to the relief of the audience—and perhaps to many of the dogs as well.

Many legendary dogfights took place before my time. But not all of them.

On that quiet spring afternoon, on a day when all the elements of the universe seemed in order, a Supai dogfight of epic proportions swept through the streets of the village. The people talk about it still—and I was there.

It started when two of the larger, more powerful mutts got into an argument over something—a bone or scrap of meat, perhaps. Once the small, isolated battle began, it rapidly drew in all dogs anywhere near the initial confrontation. Rather than moving aside to let the combatants go it alone, Supai dogs would always join a fight when it entered their terrain; hence, soon five, then ten dogs were part of the open-ended conflict of writhing bodies and slashing teeth. Like a chain reaction, within moments there were forty to fifty different animals entwined in a furious mass of flesh, totally controlling the cafeteria entrance. And the number kept growing, with more and more joining the fray. In an instant it was huge.

Now a whirlwind of activity with separate battles on the periphery, the fight moved slowly across the earth like a giant amoeba. Its random direction gave no relief to any obstacle in its path. Like a primal beast with its own inherent will, it meandered around the village kicking up breath-choking clouds of dust as it progressed.

Moving from the cafeteria to the dusty street beyond, it wound between the cottonwoods and up toward the school. Even the rustling of leaves seemed to stop with its approach. It slipped through the gate guarding the general store and flowed toward the entrance. Nothing could stand in its way. Trash cans were violently overturned. The makeshift bench came crashing to the ground. And from the midst of this giant, bizarre mass of fur and dust came the awful sounds of growling, snarling, yelping, howling, on a scale beyond belief.

When the whirlwind reached category five velocity, life in the village came to a halt. No one tried to stop the fight—that would be utterly senseless and quite dangerous. If it had been defused when only a few dogs were involved, there may have been hope. But when it reached this size and intensity, the villagers knew there was nothing to do but stand back and let it happen.

And get out of the way. All around the village center, people scattered from their places. Children were snatched up by relatives and rushed into the cafeteria, which because of its thick wooden doors—now shut tight—seemed the safest place to be. Men jumped on their horses and rode them out of harm's way. The elders previously on the bench hurried into the confines of the store. From a safe distance, people wondered which way the volatile mass would turn next. With sufficient warning, they could move in time to avoid being swept into the battle. But they had to watch it closely every minute to try to predict its movement.

The dogfight continued for what seemed like an eternity. Then suddenly something changed. At first, a few small dogs and larger ones with lethal injuries began limping away from the whirling mass. Then in a reverse chain reaction, more and more made a similar retreat for the sake of survival.

Leaving the core of dust and blood, animals staggered to the safety of the creek to wash their wounds. Others unable to walk away lay panting on the ground and let the battle move on over them. Blood stained the earth. Bits of fur and flesh were everywhere. Fierce growls were replaced by pitiful whines from participants with enough strength left to voice their pain. Almost as rapidly as it had ignited, the fiery battle burned itself out.

Soon only three or four dogs were left, fighting furiously and tiring quickly. Then there were two. Finally, the last challenger slunk away, leaving only one behind. He might have been declared a winner—but in such a contest there was no winner. Even for the victor, and most certainly for all the vanquished, weeks and weeks would pass before their wounds were healed.

The entire battle had lasted less than ten minutes. But for that brief time, life in the village stopped. Sudden and powerful, the fight had taken over events of the day and made life stand still, frozen in time until the confrontation had run its natural course.

The canine combatants limped off to nurse their wounds. Some would die, slowly or quickly, from the onslaught; others would be crippled. None would be ready for another Supai dogfight for a long time to come. Soon after the last dog crawled homeward, the dust settled, the people went back to their business, and the quiet spring afternoon returned to the canyon floor.

Flynn's Wake

My years of living closely with Indian people taught me many lessons. I learned about the land, how it changes and flows with the seasons. I learned about survival of the spirit and body under often harsh circumstances, and how laughter and the joy of being alive are tools for that survival. Most of all, I learned about interconnections in the universe, which were very different from those I learned as a child.

One such lesson was about the unequivocal reality of phenomena that cannot be explained by normal senses. Lately, a regard for such things has left the realm of sideshows, visionaries, and *Ripley's Believe It or Not* to move into the world of scientific exploration, intellectual inquiry, and even government-sponsored research. The link between prayer and healing, for example, has been studied by the Centers for Disease Control.

But to the Indian consciousness, such phenomena are not para-normal at all. To the contrary, they are simply part of the experience of living. They are not spoken of in terms of "premonition," "clairvoy-ance," or "precognition." I don't think Indian languages even have equivalent words. Rather, individual (and sometimes tribal) powers of perception extending beyond the five senses are an integral part of what it is to be a person living in harmony with the universe.

At the core of that acceptance is the traditional native view that all things of the universe are of the same spiritual substance—interchangeable, constantly evolving, fluid. Trees, rocks, clouds, animals, man, the spirit world are all interconnected, responsible to one another and dependent on deep cosmic interrelationships. Because this relationship with the universe is considered a solid truth, it is only natural that individuals can sense instantaneously events occurring in places physically far removed, and that dreamworlds and separate realities can coexist with the more familiar, often mundane reality through which we wander most of our days.

I learned this from living with Indians. And I distinctly remember the incidents that taught it to me.

I spent two years living on the Hualapai Indian Reservation just west of Grand Canyon National Park. That tribe's most closely related group, the Havasupai, live along a fertile streambed deep in the lateral recesses of the great canyon. Travel between the two main villages— Peach Springs on the Hualapai Reservation and Supai down in the canyon—was long and arduous, involving a sixty-mile dirt road to the canyon rim, and then another nine-mile switchback trail passable only by horseback or on foot. In winter and during spring thaws, the trip was often impossible.

In my time there, the phone system between the villages was archaic. A single line connected the two population centers, and almost anything could put it out of operation—the wind, an early frost, even a raven sitting on the wire winding its way down the canyon walls.

With some frequency, I would receive news that a Havasupai tribal member had just died in the Indian hospital in Phoenix and that I should notify the family, living deep in the canyon. From my trailer in Peach Springs, I would try to telephone them. But more often than not, the line was inoperative. So by shortwave radio I would contact a similar unit at the home of the physician's assistant in Supai village. The medic who answered would tell me that the family was already at his house, fully aware of the death of their relative and inquiring about funeral arrangements.

As time passed, this happened so frequently that I ceased to think of it as a chance occurrence. Somehow, the Supai family—isolated and hundreds of miles from the hospital in Phoenix—knew the instant that a loved one left their world. It simply happened that way, and I came to respect its reality.

And then there was old Flynn. Old Flynn Watahomigie was an elder of the Havasupai Nation. When I knew him, he was approaching his ninety-seventh year—a full life for an amazing man. Flynn was one of the last in the line of traditional Havasupai chiefs. The position had been passed on from generation to generation within certain clans, for it was known that such families held chief's blood whereas others were healers and still others carried on the tradition of rainmaking. The line was broken in the mid-1940s when the government-mandated tribal-chairman-and-council model was forced on the Havasupai and an "elected" official was installed in the chief's place.

Even so, Flynn carried the blood of chiefs in his lineage. He was deeply respected among his people, not only for his ancestry but also for his wisdom and character.

He was a small and wiry man, active until a few months before his death, when the pressures of ninety-seven years finally took their toll. By then, he had sired eight children—the youngest, a son born when Flynn was eighty-five. He was a proud father and spent much time teaching his children in the ways of survival. He demanded that they learn the duality of knowledge to help them exist in a world no longer Indian. They were schooled in traditional ways as well as in book knowledge and English.

In his younger years, Flynn lived with the Havasupai. He worked horses and mules every day, bringing supplies from the rim down the difficult trail into Supai village. In the harsh winter months, he and his family lived above the canyon on the plateau, where food and firewood were more plentiful. In summer, they returned to their small home on the canyon floor, where he irrigated his crops of melons, corn, and beans with water from the Havasu Creek. Life in those days was always busy.

In his later years, Flynn moved from the canyon to Peach Springs, to be with relatives. He married a Hualapai women thirty years his junior, produced strong children, and stayed in that more cosmopolitan village until his death. Life in Hualapai land was equally busy as he worked the small herds of cattle and horses and built addition after addition on the family home.

I remember Flynn coming regularly to the clinic in the months before his death. The visits pleased him. He enjoyed telling me old stories and was amused by my frustration at not being able to alter the inevitable course of his last days. He always had a twinkle in his eye. I'd give him a little something here for arthritis, a bit of something else for a urinary infection. We would visit for long periods and speak of things—the weather, his horses, the future of his people.

Flynn knew he was dying and that his time was near. There was no fear or sadness in his spirit, for he had lived a full and powerful life and believed deeply in the continuing cycles of birth, death, and rebirth. Preparing himself, he would gather his children, singularly or in groups, and repeat again important lessons he wanted to pass on. In addition, he would instruct them not to be saddened by his leaving.

Then one day Flynn made the journey from this world to another. It happened quietly at home. It was like the frosted breath of a horse in winter, or a gentle southern breeze rising from the canyon. It was a whisper.

As was the tradition with the Hualapai and Havasupai, a community wake, or "sing," would be held for the old man. Such sings had been held for centuries, and although there were now a few modern influences—such as expensive caskets and store-bought gifts for the participants—the old songs, feelings, and spirituality remained intact. The body would be brought to the community center, where everyone would gather and mourn. Ancient chants, prayers, and dances would go on through the night. The women would wail while the men drummed and danced.

The dull gray walls of the community center would be transformed by hundreds of men, women, and children. The hypnotic rhythm of drums and chants would assert itself, capturing the moment. Bodies would sway in unison. Eulogies and prayers would be offered to the departed soul. Hour after hour the energy level would build, and no one in attendance—Indian or non-Indian—would be able to doubt the sense of things beyond.

Tradition called for the sing to last as long as it took to prepare the tribal member for the "journey" from one reality to another. The more powerful and respected the member, the more intense the sing must be. Sings would last anywhere from twelve hours to days, depending on what needed to be accomplished to continue the life cycle.

Flynn's sing would, of course, be an especially powerful one. His bloodline and the fullness of his life demanded it. A great deal of collective energy was therefore needed to prepare Flynn for his journey.

The family brought his body to the community center in late afternoon. Traditional meals were prepared, and villagers began gathering. Many Havasupai families had traveled long miles to Peach Springs to add their tribute. But for some reason, by early evening the community center was only partially full. Not enough people were there to begin the sing.

Everyone was still *planning* to attend—there was no question about that. But with finishing the evening meal, feeding horses, tending to family chores, visiting with Havasupai friends, maybe even waiting for a television show to end, many had yet to head for the community center. Whatever the reason, the crowd was surprisingly small for Flynn's sing, not at all proper for such a powerful occasion.

Suddenly, about eight o'clock, every light in the village went out. Televisions went blank. The darkness was total. Peach Springs underwent a total electrical blackout.

I, too, was behind schedule that night. I remember walking outside my trailer when the power failed. A near-full moon dominated the cloudless sky and illuminated the earth with a subtle, eerie radiance. The entire village spread out below me, but not a light could be seen. The silence was thunderous, overwhelming. People drifted out of their homes, looking about at the sky, the moon, and the darkness.

I felt something in the moment. It was not a spirit of hostility or evil. Something, however, was present, and it touched everyone in the village that night.

Standing on my ridge, I slowly realized what was happening. The villagers below had sensed it immediately. Their presence was being "requested" at the community center to show proper respect for the old chief. The cold and the moon and the illuminated earth spoke of only one thing: for all tribal members to assemble so the sing could begin.

Before driving down to join them, I called the electric company in Kingman, some sixty miles to the west. They promised to send someone out immediately to fix the blackout. About thirty minutes later, with the center packed and the chanting in full force, the lights returned as abruptly as they had failed. But the repair crew was still driving in from the west. There had been no time for checks or repairs.

Later, the repair foreman was at a loss to explain why the power had failed. All lines were intact, all terminals were fine, no circuit breakers or transformer switches had flipped. Everything was normal, the utility man told me, and the blackout could not be explained by equipment failure.

But to those of us in the village that night, the reason for it was obvious. Flynn Watahomigie required all the energy of the tribe to send him on his way. A big crowd was needed. So Flynn simply gathered the crowd.

Robinson

 THE FIRST TIME I SAW ROBINSON, I was struck by his physical presence in the crowd at a basketball game. Sitting in the bleachers in that small community gymnasium, he immediately captured the eye. Mysterious, even a bit dangerous.

I came to know this young man for a brief time during the years I spent living with the Hualapai Indian people. The Hualapais are a relatively unknown band, except in Arizona, where they are sometimes called "them people up north." About 3,000 strong, they live on a wedge-shaped reservation of almost a million acres of strikingly beautiful land along the Grand Canyon's south rim. It is their ancestral land, the place where they have always been. Its high-desert plains, pine-covered mountains, and deep, angular canyons leading down to the Colorado River are the context in which the collective history of these people has always taken place.

Robinson was three-fourths Hualapai by heritage. The other quarter of his "blood quorum" was Apache. He was between twenty and twenty-three years old, just entering the prime of young adulthood.

Around the reservation his appearance was immediately recognized as different. Most Hualapai people are short, a bit rotund, with broad, smiling faces. Robinson, having inherited an extra dose of genes from the pool of his Apache ancestors, was exactly the opposite. He was tall, more than six feet, with an angular, lanky body. His face was strikingly handsome with classic features: a thin jaw line, high cheekbones, a sharply angled nose, and deep, penetrating black eyes. His complexion was clear and rich; its hue mirrored the red rocks of those canyon lands. His black, silky hair, in the traditional long style, fell almost to the middle of his back.

Robinson had recently returned to the reservation after several years away at schools and in urban areas. He had grown up with the Hualapais, but there had seemingly always been some tension because of his mixed-blood status. He never fit into the young-boy social strata in that small village and was often the butt of jokes and gossip. Instead of being educated in the village, he had been sent away to boarding schools for both his elementary and high school training. After finishing school in Phoenix, he stayed a long time in that city hundreds of miles to the south. Talk was that he then lived a few years with distant relatives in California. Middle-aged people around the village muttered that he had become very much the "urban Indian," a thinly veiled put-down of someone who felt superior to his reservation counterparts.

He had returned about a year earlier and was, like many young men in the village, simply hanging around much of the time. Occasionally, he worked at seasonal tribal jobs on land management or forest fire suppression. Most of the time, however, he spent hours each day at the community center, general store, and gas station with the other out-of-work young men.

Since returning to the village, Robinson had become an unlikely hero to those men. He had a captivating personality—often quiet and mysterious, yet spellbinding on those rare occasions when he spoke. During his time in cities, he had developed a deep pride in his Indian heritage and a militant arrogance toward the dominant white society that had perpetrated such horrors on native peoples throughout the hemisphere. He had also taken part in the Indian political movements that were sweeping the country. Centered in urban settings, the movements had not yet filtered down to the reservation with the intensity that Robinson had experienced.

So he would tell the young men in the village of his newfound pride and anger. He would speak to them of AIM, the American Indian Movement, and of confrontations with guns in South Dakota. They, in response, would speak of tribal history now almost lost to remembrance—the healing ceremonies, the religious rites, the language and songs. As they spoke of the losses, their anger grew and solidified.

When the talk wasn't political, it focused on two equally important issues: rock 'n' roll and basketball. Robinson loved music, and had even learned some electric guitar back in California. He and his friends would listen to heavy metal rock 'n' roll by the hour, with the stereo cranked up to thunderous levels. Music became the anthem of their movement, its battle cry for the days to come: Led Zeppelin, the Rolling Stones, and an all-Indian group called XIT.

And basketball. Basketball to the young men represented a perfect blend of a team sport where people worked together (as in the tribe) and where the true beauty of individual magic could also occur. It didn't require the equipment or space necessary for football. The ground was too rocky and dusty for baseball. But any slab of concrete with a basket at the end would do for a quick pickup game. And the community center had two good hardwood courts where most village life centered from November through the spring thaws. Basketball was more than a pastime for Robinson and his crowd; it was a religious undertaking. They would play it for hours every day, and hone to a fine edge their subtle interplays of body and nonverbal awareness on the court.

They also drank together, with Robinson in the lead. Every chance they had, the group would catch a ride down old Route 66 toward the west and congregate among the bars just on the other side of the reservation line. The reservation itself was dry—no liquor was sold. But on its edge, a collection of package stores and seedy bars could be found. The young men would buy six-packs and jugs of cheap wine, and sit out back amid broken glass and old cans, drinking the days away as they talked of politics and music and their anger.

Robinson was, like most, a binge drinker. He would sometimes stay drunk for days at a time. I would often see him during those binges, for he would come to the clinic whenever the pain of drinking forced him to seek help. But Robinson also had long periods when drinking was not relevant. It was during those times that his strength and charisma were most obvious. His eyes were clear and sparkled as he talked of his dreams. His warrior side was in full bloom. But there was always an undercurrent of danger and fear—much like that appearing in the eyes of a trapped wild animal.

We saw each other a lot in those days. I ran the four-room clinic in the village, and my government-issue residential trailer was next door. After-hours, people needing to see the doctor would come straight to the trailer. All through the evening and night, the door would explode with loud raps—from parents with sick children, drunks home from a fight, and people in pain of spirit.

Robinson often came by during those off-hours. Sometimes he had been drinking, but often, especially as time went on and our friendship grew, he came by just to talk and look at my books. And since my stereo was one of the most powerful in the village, he would sit for hours listening to music on my headphones. Little substantial talk took place between us in the beginning.

But as time went on, a certain cautious friendship developed. We shared a love of basketball and music. I was enthralled and moved by his reports of the growing political element among Indians throughout cities and reservations. He told me of their plans, their struggles; I told him of my personal journey from the rigid, numbing technology of East Coast existence to an understanding of his people's healing ways. Modern medicine, for me, had become a charade that merely covered the wounds and numbed the pain instead of restoring the balance that had been disrupted. We became hesitant allies in our individual wanderings, and we learned much from each other during that time.

In autumn of that year, things suddenly changed for Robinson. Those of us who knew him well were the first to notice the subtle, and then more obvious signs of a growing disharmony in his spirit. For a number of weeks I didn't see him around the village. There was talk that he had gone back to Phoenix or California. Nobody was sure, for he had spoken to no one before leaving. He had simply disappeared.

When he returned, his withdrawal was apparent to all. He stopped working for tribal business and no longer hung out at the gas station. He came to my trailer a few times, always drunk, and our interchanges were unfortunate. He was always looking for a handout or wanting to get into an argument about the white man and what "my people" had done to his collective Indian identity. Seeing him approach the trailer became so troublesome that I dreaded our interactions.

Our last visit was on a bright weekend in early October. Although the evenings were crisp with fall air, the days were still delightfully warm and clear. I was working out behind the trailer on a makeshift horse corral I had fashioned out of old railroad ties and warped boards. Robinson came bouncing over the fence, clear-eyed and smiling broadly.

His greeting and mood were upbeat—a distinct change from the Robinson of previous weeks. We spoke about the day and how the rangy tribal cattle stock were beginning to show thick coats of winter fur. We compared the prospects for various basketball teams in the upcoming season. We shared easy and happy things that warm October day.

As our talk softened, Robinson began speaking of ancestral matters. He described his traditional views of how the Great Spirit was found in all things—people, rocks, wind, the animals, and spirit forms. He spoke of the passage of energy back and forth between all interconnected elements of Earth and Sky. He spoke gently about freedom of spirit. He seemed strong, committed. The bright sun illuminated his face, and the breeze fanned out his black hair into a majestic lion's mane.

The next day I was busy at the clinic, seeing scores of patients with problems that had developed over the weekend. Just past lunchtime, I got a call from the Highway Patrol dispatcher in Kingman—there had been a "pedestrian–motor vehicle encounter" near the small border town just west of the reservation.

Such calls for emergency assistance came straight to the clinic, since our aging carryall van served as the only ambulance within sixty miles; and as the only doctor within that same radius, I was often both driver and technician. I grabbed my emergency bag and keys to the ambulance, then yelled to our custodian to jump in and help me.

We sped down Route 66 to the west. Route 66, the legendary main road to the California coast, led right through the village and the reservation. It was an old, two-lane highway that had fallen into disrepair as the new interstate neared completion ten miles to the south. But at that time, 66 was still heavily traveled by cars, motor homes, and semitrailers, all speeding west toward Las Vegas or east toward Albuquerque. Accidents were common, especially on bitter winter nights when treacherous ice patches formed. As the only medically trained people around, we responded, but we had neither the equipment nor the expertise to handle things well.

The custodian and I drove in silence as we monitored the radio information between the police and their dispatcher. I felt a sickness inside. These calls for crisis emergency care were always difficult and draining. It was a frequent phenomenon that local people, staggeringly drunk, would leave the bars and begin wandering toward their homes in the village. Their unsteadiness and the speeding trucks often made a critical connection there on Route 66. The results were always tragic.

I sensed from static-filled reports that the police decided a doctor was not really needed. "He looks dead to me," someone said. I felt an uncomfortable ambivalence. At least I wouldn't have to spend the next four hours providing critical care to a badly traumatized patient as we covered the sixty miles to the hospital in Kingman. But it would be another tragic event collectively experienced by tribal members, for everyone at Hualapai knew everyone else, and a sudden death like this would touch them all and only reaffirm the misery felt by these people.

We were almost at the accident site, so I sped on. Three or four police cars with flashing lights were alongside the road. Traffic was being slowly directed through the area, as tourists and truckers strained to stare. A few officers and bystanders were gathered ten feet away from an angular mass covered by a white plastic sheet, lying in the rough sagebrush just off the road. I walked up, nodded hello to the tribal and state policemen, and asked what had happened.

The story was familiar. This trucker, they said while pointing to a man nervously smoking a cigarette down the road, was traveling west when some fool Indian just seemed to jump in front of his rig. No time to react. It was over in an instant.

There was something different about this story. Usually, the victim was seen walking in the middle of the road, or staggering, or doing something to indicate alcohol had taken over their functioning. But the trucker swore the Indian had shown no such signs. He was standing along the road, and then suddenly flung himself in the truck's path.

Once or twice a year we would experience a similar event. Not the action of a drunk, but a conscious suicide. It was a local pattern. The trucks speeding through reservation land were a quick, effective, and demonstrative means of bringing an end to the suffering of spirit. Other tribes had different mechanisms, I had been told. Some Apache bands were apt to use rifles. Other groups would cut their wrists or take an overdose.

As the sheet was pulled back, I walked over to the body. Somehow, I felt no shock or surprise when I looked down on the still, unsoiled face of Robinson. His body was twisted horribly from the sudden impact at sixty miles per hour, but his face was clear and untouched. A little dirt was in his hair, yet otherwise he had the quiet face of someone asleep.

I drove back to the village in silence. Many thoughts came, and went, and returned again. Robinson was the village's third young person I had known who had committed suicide that year. The youth, the power and hope of the tribe, were being whittled away by this impoverishment of spirit. There seemed to be no answers for them or, at the moment, for me. Only sadness and loss. I didn't cry—I couldn't—for my tears had been drained by the previous tragedies.

I parked in front of the clinic and walked north to a piñon-covered expanse leading down toward the canyon. The sky was cloudless.

Deep blue, no sounds except an occasional caw of ravens as they circled overhead. A soft breeze began to sway the squat pines.

So utterly beautiful, I thought. I tried to let the perfect order of that earth and sky bring some measure of peace to the pain inside. But still, I felt such sadness for what had just happened.

Suddenly, a small whirl of wind and dust kicked up about forty yards in front of me. It quickly grew in intensity, and I recognized it as one of the small, mysterious "dust devils" that occasionally formed over open spaces when the right combination of heat and wind produced those short-lived tornadoes. It grew and grew in height. Yet unlike most dust devils, this one seemed not to be moving laterally. Its small tip bit at the ground, raising light-brown plumes of dust toward the sky. It was a strange dust devil, different from any I had ever seen.

I looked upward toward its ever rising cone. There, perhaps 100 feet above the earth, balanced perfectly in the air, was an indistinct black object. It seemed at first like a piece of roofing tar paper or an old box that had been lifted by the little cyclone. But as I kept looking, its form became more and more amorphous. It floated and soared. It rose higher and higher.

The visible signs of the whirling devil soon disappeared. No more rising dust or breezes striking my face. No sounds. The only presence was that dark object, now rising to 200, then 300 feet into the clearness of sky. It rose with an incredible speed. I watched it go on and on, until the eye could not discern it anymore. It was swallowed into the heavens.

I knew at once that it was Robinson on his passage. It wasn't an intellectual conclusion, for surely my logic would not accept such an event. It was a deep, inherent sense of what I had witnessed. It was as true as any truth in my experience.

Robinson's spirit had found its freedom. The necessary passage from one form into another, to join the Great Spirit's presence in all things, had taken place for him. For whatever reasons Robinson had not found harmony in his human form, the skies now claimed him. And he was flying, free and strong.

An overwhelming peacefulness came to me. I smiled, then began laughing out loud into the sky.

I heard a call from behind me at the clinic. Come on, it said loudly, there are people waiting to be seen. Are you coming back in now?

I took one last look at the sky, turned, and went back to work.

Birth Story

TO MOST PEOPLE, the training of a physician is a mystery. Even those with pride in their awareness think that somehow doctors are ready-made doctors, coming off medical-school assembly lines like new cars rolling down ramps in Detroit or Tokyo—fully equipped and functional, aware of and able to treat all the afflictions besetting humankind.

Not so, of course. The young person just graduated from medical school, despite the MD after the name, is full of scientific knowledge but ever so short on experience. Only time and exposure to the endless variation of physical problems can bring that essential element of becoming a competent and caring physician.

Take the delivery of babies, for example. Most medical students' experience with the infinite possibilities of this natural process consists of a basic four- to six-week clinical rotation early in their training. Only those specializing in obstetrics or family practice confront the complexity of the rare and crucial problems that may arise during birth.

Giving birth. The ultimate experience for most women—and increasingly, for men assisting in the process. Those present can watch the painful yet joyous expressions, the blood and secretions, the first gasp of breath in new life—all magic sensations at the core of our human journey.

Early in my career as a physician, two birth adventures taught me that things are not always as they seem—that despite my wealth of knowledge, I had much to learn.

I had recently arrived to work in the small, isolated Indian village of Peach Springs. Located on old Route 66 in northern Arizona, Peach Springs was the population center for the Hualapai Indian Nation, a band of 3,000 souls living on their traditional lands abutting the Grand Canyon's southern rim.

I was as fresh and squeaky-clean as a new physician could be. I had completed four years at a prestigious Eastern medical school, then taken a one-year internship at a large community hospital north of Philadelphia. The internship was one of the last classic "rotating" programs, an intense year of exposure to a variety of specialties—pediatrics, internal medicine, surgery, psychiatry, obstetrics, emergency medicine. I was not yet drawn toward any particular specialty, and felt that this smorgasbord of experience would lead me in more defined directions.

All the internship did, however, was further confuse my path. I was drained from the long hours and intensity of managing so many sick patients at once. Any thought of continuing the pace for another four years of residency was out of the question. But no alternative seemed clear.

This was in the late 1960s, the time of Vietnam. Although the unpopular war was in its last throes, President Nixon was attempting to cut his losses and bomb the North Vietnamese "back to the stone age." As a newly trained physician with eight years of educational deferment, I was swimming on top of the big draft pool. I had been publicly opposed to the war for seven years and had been involved in marches to Washington, sit-ins, and other demonstrations throughout the country with people who simply said, "This is insane. I will not participate."

It wasn't the danger of war that I opposed. Nor the discomfort of being uprooted from a comfortable existence and forced to wear the same underwear for weeks at a time. I admired the tens of thousands of men and women who had volunteered and served without complaint during those horrible years. I was more than willing to do my part for the country's responsibility to the world, no matter how harsh the sacrifice.

But serving in war had become tantamount to rejecting all I believed in. At first, I was opposed only to the Vietnam War and its mirroring of both our perverse paranoia of Communism and our complete misreading of Third World peoples. Then as my personal commitment matured, I realized that I was, at my core, a pacifist. Using the force of armaments and destruction to reach political and economic goals had become, for me, a nonviable solution. I could not serve that effort.

It was during my internship that I became aware of the US Public Health Service, a little-known branch of government that provided health-care personnel for a wide variety of entities—the federal prison system, Coast Guard, National Institutes of Health, Centers for Disease Control, to name a few. And one small piece of that large pie was Indian Health Service (IHS), a group mandated to care for Indian people across the country as promised through treaty and trust agreements.

I had been developing a budding interest in Indian people at about the same time. Growing up on the East Coast, I had only a woefully naive exposure to Indians, based primarily on living in a town named after Hiawatha's mother and cheering for the Washington Redskins. But then one evening, while lying horizontal in the intern's on-call room after forty-eight hours of constant work, I found myself numbly watching a Public Broadcasting television special on the Oglala Sioux in South Dakota. What I saw were not noble savages or cartoon profiles on football helmets, but rather abject poverty, ramshackle homes unable to keep out winter chill, drunken men staggering down dusty roads, and pain in children's faces. I wanted to learn more about this paradox.

At the same time, the unanswered questions in my life seemed to be falling together, as if the cosmos were clicking in tune with itself. I applied for the Public Health Service and was accepted as a commissioned officer, thereby negating the necessity to either flee to Canada or accept a jail term for refusing the draft. I asked to be assigned to Indian Health Service, so that I might serve a people who sorely needed the help after having given up so much to the more aggressive American society.

It all happened quickly and without a hitch. Two days after finishing my internship in June 1972, I loaded my van with virtually all my possessions and headed west across the great expanse of land to assume my first official IHS assignment—running the small outpatient clinic in Peach Springs, Arizona.

The clinic had four small examination rooms, an antiquated X-ray machine, and a small pharmacy. The nearest general hospital was in Kingman, sixty miles to the west. The closest Indian hospital, intended to serve as an inpatient facility for the Hualapais, was almost 120 miles to the southwest, in Parker, Arizona.

Babies had traditionally been born at home on the reservation up until the early 1960s. But as the IHS system became more developed, strong pressure was placed on Hualapai mothers to have their babies in a hospital setting. Prenatal care would be provided at the Peach Springs clinic for the first eight months, then as the mother's due date approached, she was strongly encouraged to take the long journey to Parker and sit patiently around the hospital—far from home and family—to wait until labor began. The hospital in Kingman was used only for sudden, unexpected births, and the IHS system frowned on its regular use by Hualapai mothers, because of limited funds to pay for their care. Those unfortunate women with high-risk pregnancies were often flown to the tertiary Indian medical center in Phoenix for an even more extended stay before delivery.

It was a system devised to provide what IHS thought was a safe, medically appropriate way to reverse the distressing rates of infant mortality on the reservation. At the time, there was neither awareness of nor appreciation for home birthing as a viable alternative. Few children were born at home anymore. And with the nearest hospital sixty miles away and poorly equipped for severe obstetric problems, this plan seemed the most practical solution to a difficult situation.

It was all for the best, I felt, as I began my first few months operating that isolated clinic. My skills in childbirth were not extensive. I had gone through the requisite clinical rotation early in medical school, then spent another four weeks on an obstetric service during my internship, but my role in those births was mainly that of an observer. There was always close supervision and rarely was I faced with making independent decisions. It was one of the many areas of medicine in which I felt inadequate. Although part of me regretted that the young women had to separate themselves from family and culture during those weeks of waiting in Parker, I suspected they were better off than in my inexperienced hands.

My beliefs changed one evening a few months after I began living with the Hualapais. I was just finishing an early dinner when a knock came at the door of my trailer next to the clinic. A Hualapai man stood outside. He appeared frightened and out of breath. "Come quickly," he said. "We need help at the house. It's my wife."

I jumped in the old clinic ambulance and followed his pickup truck over dusty roads through the hillsides south of the village. It was an area of the reservation I had not yet seen, away from the central village, which had electricity and running water. The light of sunset was rapidly fading, and the dust kicked up by his truck made it difficult to see the irregular road before me.

We finally arrived at a weathered, single-room shack nestled against a small hill. A few cars and trucks were parked outside. A group of men stood silently by a pickup. I could see an outdoor privy slightly down the hill and a tall stack of firewood alongside it. A pack of mongrel dogs barked incessantly as I hopped from the ambulance and followed the man up the shaky wooden steps to the house. He stayed outside, motioning for me to walk in.

The one large room was bathed in the soft glow of kerosene

lamps and propane lanterns. Otherwise, it was a typical Hualapai family dwelling—neat yet packed to the ceiling with the collective possessions of an extended family. Many cots could be seen around the perimeter of the room. A large wooden table occupied the center, and off to the side I could see an area for food preparation, although there was no water faucet.

At the back of the room I noticed a young woman lying under a mound of blankets, her head and back propped up by pillows. She was moaning softly. A number of middle-aged and older women stood beside her, wiping her brow and comforting her in the guttural native language of the Hualapai.

I walked over and sat on the edge of the cot. The young woman's face was so youthful, almost like that of a teenager. She appeared frightened, and steady beads of sweat formed on her forehead. Her hands were clasped around her lower abdomen, and even through the heavy blankets that covered her I could see the distended abdomen of a woman about to have a baby.

One of the older women, whom I recognized from clinic visits, softly informed me of the situation. This was the girl's first baby, and she wasn't supposed to be due for another month. She had had only one prenatal visit to the clinic, about seven months ago, before I arrived in the village. She had been doing well, so the family felt no pressure to bring her for follow-up visits. Anyway, the clinic was for sick people, not those who felt fine, the woman explained.

The young woman had begun cramping six hours earlier and had passed some fluid and blood about two hours ago. The cramps were now frequent and intense, the women in attendance said. There had been some thought to rush her by pickup to the hospital in Kingman, but they had decided there was not enough time. Besides, they said, those white people at the Kingman hospital always treat Indians badly. They make you wait and don't pay any attention. And they are always asking if they will get paid.

I laid back the blankets and touched the young woman's distended abdomen with my slightly tremulous hands. She began to cry quietly when a contraction began, and I measured its duration and intensity as I had been taught in medical school. It was a major, effective contraction, and within a minute of the muscles relaxing, another two-minute contraction kicked in. Noticing a steady flow of blood-tinged mucus and fluid from between her legs, I held off examining her vagina for the moment. There was no doubt she was in active labor and the birth was imminent.

I tried to be reassuring, but my mind was racing. What was I to do? I was the doctor, of course, but I didn't feel versed enough in any of this. Should I try to help her here on the cot or should I attempt to get her in the ambulance and back to the clinic, where I had more equipment, water, and light? What if there were problems—a breech, an arrested labor, uncontrolled hemorrhaging? Possibilities rushed through my head as the young woman again moaned and a propane lamp near my head hissed with its soft flame. I felt momentarily paralyzed.

I hurried out to the ambulance and retrieved a makeshift obstetrical kit that had been gathering dust on the shelf. The kit had been sealed tight months before, and I had never looked inside to see what equipment it held. Returning to the bedside, I began to prepare the area. I then opened the kit and laid out various supplies next to the cot.

The women were calm and helpful, giving instructions to the young woman and comforting her during the contractions. Their reassurances steadied my frenzied nerves as well. I became more confident and internally returned to a place where the business at hand took precedence over the fear of possible problems. As I examined the laboring woman more closely and felt the baby's head almost ready to emerge, the others kept speaking softly about how well things were going, how everything was going to be fine.

I felt as though their collective experience of childbirth was guiding me that evening. They gave me the illusion of being in control, but in actuality, I was simply following their suggestions, which were tempered by time and history. No longer was I shaking. It was a walk in the park.

The baby came quickly and easily. He was small—perhaps five

or six pounds—but a good baby. He burst forth with a hearty cry as soon as the body was delivered. After clamping and cutting the umbilical cord, I gave the baby to the women, who cleaned and warmed him in fresh blankets of multicolored wool. I observed as the women took him off to a corner of the room and performed a traditional anointing. All the while, a soft Indian song filled the small room, providing a counterpoint to the glowing lanterns.

The mother appeared to be doing fine. The contractions had lessened, and no serious bleeding was occurring. The placenta delivered a short time later, and I could see no troublesome tears or injuries from the birth.

Someone in the family said they would take the woman and baby to the Kingman hospital that evening—"just to be checked." I concurred, but secretly knew they would not go. Babies had been born in that shack for generations, and those women knew when things were fine. In any case, I promised to see the mother and baby at the clinic the next day.

I stepped out into the nighttime air and joined the collection of men by the pickup. There were smiles all around and teasing slaps on the back of the young father. Many of their comments were in Hualapai, but the message was clear.

That crisp fall evening had turned to night, countless stars filled the sky, and sounds of large owls on their nightly hunts could be heard from over the hills. I made one last stop inside the shack to check on mother and baby. The women were trading old and new stories, all with laughter and smiles. The young woman was sipping a homemade broth, and the infant was suckling voraciously. The women kept telling me how well it had gone and what a fine doctor I was. I felt embarrassed, for I knew I had done little. It was they who had led me through the process—one that had taken place among Hualapai women for centuries. I just happened to be around for that one.

My other birth story, although less successful, was still thunderous in its lessons. About a month later, a knock came on the door after-hours. On the porch of my trailer stood a Hualapai man in his mid-thirties. I had seen him around the village and knew his mother well, for she made frequent trips to the clinic as we monitored her diabetes. I didn't know the man's name, though we had exchanged brief greetings in the past. I invited him in, but he politely refused, saying he did not want to track mud in the trailer. I looked at his weathered cowboy boots, which were covered to above the ankles with a thick, reddish earth. His old jeans and denim jacket were similarly muddy, and he wore a thin yellow rain slicker. He took off his sweat-soaked tan cowboy hat and held it in both hands at his front, as if presenting himself at a reception.

Could I come help him with a medical problem? he asked haltingly. He seemed embarrassed, but pressed on. It was unusual, he said, but his father thought I might be of help. Slowly, he described how one of their cattle was giving birth down in the canyon, but had developed a complication. The birth was incomplete, he said. The calf was stuck and they all felt sure the cow would die unless something could be done. Could I just come by and look?

In that village, the clinic doctor inevitably faced a twin role: caring for human needs, of course, yet also being available to double as a veterinarian, since the nearest vet was sixty miles to the west. I had been told by the previous clinic physician that I might be approached about sick animals, and although he had been hesitant to accept such appeals, the choice was up to me. Having grown up in the suburbs, I was inexperienced at watching the birth of farm animals, much less "doctoring" range stock. But since the anatomy and physiology of all mammals are somewhat similar, I figured, maybe I can be of help.

I knew that Hualapai cattle were a lifeblood of the depressed reservation economy. The million-plus reservation acres provided a sparse but reasonable grazing area for cattle, and hundreds of head roamed the land. Some were owned by individual families; many others were owned collectively by the tribe. Although life for cattle on the reservation was a delicate balance of survival, the loss of a breeding cow could be devastating to a family that relied on cattle raising as its principal means of income. Of course I had to go see if I could be of help.

I gathered a few supplies from the clinic and jumped in the Jeep that was part of the three-vehicle government motor pool. Although rain was not falling in the village, I could see dark clouds and sheets of heavy rain to the north, in the lateral canyons that drained into the Colorado River.

I followed the man's pickup truck down a rock-strewn trail paralleling one of the canyons. The evening light was failing rapidly. Lightning flashed frequently to the north, and the wind came up cold and damp. The Jeep lurched forward and the gearbox whined as the wheels grabbed hold of muddy depressions and bumped over large boulders in the road.

After forty minutes, we arrived on a plateau at the northwest end of the reservation. I had not been to that area before, for it was not easily accessible. Squat piñon and juniper trees dotted the plateau. Sagebrush covered the rest of the expanse, giving an appearance of carpeting to the otherwise barren landscape.

We approached a slight rise where four pickup trucks were parked in a semicircle, all with their lights pointed toward a central area twenty feet ahead. The flood of headlights caught a fine rain falling in silvery sheets, and lightning flashed as in a strobe, all providing a mysterious, almost theatrical backdrop.

I threw on a heavy coat and joined the men standing in the rain. Lying on the wet earth was a massive cow covered with mud and pieces of sagebrush. Her large eyes were wide and filled with fear. As she panted rapidly, warm breath rose as steam from her nostrils and caught the light from the trucks. She would lie still, then suddenly lurch sideways as a moan rumbled out from deep in her chest. The strong smell of manure and other primal secretions struck me full in the face. She was the largest, scariest, most disgusting-looking creature I had ever seen.

Standing at her rear, I could see the hind end of a calf protruding from her uterus, along with two spindly legs and a thin, matted tail.

There was no spontaneous movement from the calf. As from the cow's nostrils, a fine steam also rose from her flanks, like a smoldering volcano or primal place of creation.

The men were busily working around the cow. It was obvious they were not looking to me for direction, for they knew this work far better than I. A few older men seemed mildly upset I had even been called, but I was treated reasonably by all. Little talk transpired among them as they attempted to remove the calf from its embedded position, causing the cow to buck and kick wildly. The rain increased to a downpour.

From their conversations in Hualapai and broken English, I got the gist that the calf was probably dead and their efforts were to save the cow if possible. I slowly approached the cow's flank end and touched the calf's muddy, still body. My cold, numb fingers felt only a chilling frigidity—no sense of life-sustaining warmth. I reached carefully inside the cow's vagina and felt the calf's bony chest for signs of a palpable heartbeat. The cow lay still, seemingly exhausted. The little chest gave no movement, no pulse of life.

The men decided it was time for more drastic action. They fashioned a makeshift pulley out of chains and a hand-held come-along device. One end of the chain was thrown around a sturdy juniper trunk ten feet away; the other was tied around the cow's upper quarters behind the forelegs. The cow began objecting again, this time with more uncontrolled fear. She bucked and bellowed and attempted to bite at the men fastening the chain around her chest.

A thick rope was then tied to the calf's hindquarters. I was asked to pull my Jeep up to the rear so they could utilize the electric winch on the front bumper. I suddenly realized why I had been called to help: they needed the winch, not my medical expertise. At least it was comforting to be needed for something.

With the chains and ropes securely fashioned in opposite directions, we began the extraction. The winch was engaged at a slow speed, attempting a modified "forceps" delivery of the breech calf. Horrible sounds began emanating from the cow. She kicked and attempted to rise, but was held in place by the two now-taut tethers between tree and Jeep. The calf was not moving an inch, although great spurts of blood and fluid erupted from the cow's uterus. The pain in her eyes, the smell of fresh feces and blood, the lightning flashes in the sky overhead—it was a dreamworld scene from the depths of hell, the kind of image pounded into my consciousness by the stern-faced priests of my youth.

We stopped the winch and began to rethink the process. The men talked back and forth in Hualapai, making subtle motions with their lips and hands as they devised a new plan. The Jeep was repositioned at a sharper angle from the cow, and the chains readjusted.

The winch was again engaged. The cow, mustering renewed energy from deep within, began to bellow and kick. This time we could definitely see some movement in the calf's locked position. Barely perceptible at first, the slow slide outward became more obvious within seconds. The winch was stopped, and the hand-held lever device was attached to provide greater, more subtle control over the pull. As the men began jacking the to-and-fro lever on the come-along, I positioned my hand inside the cow's vagina to assist with the delivery and perhaps prevent a full eversion of the uterus, a condition that would undoubtedly be fatal.

With little effort, we delivered the forelegs and head. The calf was withered and deformed. There was no sadness, for calves died all the time in that often hostile landscape. It was an accepted fact of the delicate nature of life.

All attention turned to the cow. She was still panting, but the fear had gone from her eyes. She was bleeding minimally, and I could detect no major injuries to her birth area. The men were pleased. She will heal herself, they said. Cows are tough.

I prepared a large syringe full of megadose antibiotics—penicillin and streptomycin—which seemingly was the cure-all for most illnesses affecting horses, cows, dogs, and other four-legged creatures. The cow did not even wince as I injected her in the thick chest muscles.

Calmness returned to that high plateau. The rains had stopped and lightning was only occasionally seen far off in the distant canyons.

There was a freshness in the air that comes after rain falls on that parched land. I passed a little time with the men in small talk. But it was after midnight, and I needed to return to Peach Springs to prepare for another full day at the clinic.

As I began to drive away, my lights caught sight of the cow, now standing and grazing actively on the sagebrush.

Two births. Two results. And many lessons learned—lessons that held me in good stead later on. I delivered a number of babies over the next two years, and each event brought more self-assurance. I often thought back to the glow of lanterns in the one-room shack and the comforting conversation of the women.

And I gained a fair reputation over those years as someone who could also doctor a horse or cow with great success. As long as I had enough thick white antibiotic solution in my back pocket, all my furry patients seemed to get better.

Such was the way in this place where birth represented a new start for all the creatures of the canyon country.

Pendleton
Roundup

"INDIANS. ATTENTION, INDIANS. We'll be ready for you in five minutes. All Indians, get ready by the gate."

Slowly the people begin to move from their weathered tepees, tall and majestic in the afternoon heat of this eastern Oregon day. Women, children, infants in arms—all emerging from the canvas-covered entranceways of their four-day makeshift homes. Their garments are magnificent and colorful. Ancestral clothing and ornaments passed down through generations are countered with new dresses and leggings of leather and beads, all in the traditional, honored method. The hot, dry afternoon comes alive with color and feathers, beads and tinkling bells, headdresses and bright shawls. The people are gathering.

From around the far end of the tepee village, near the corrals, men and boys appear on horses. Their clothing and ornaments are like those worn by the walkers. Each wide-chested Indian horse has its own beaded-and-leathered breastplate, feathered bridle, and long, brightly colored woolen blanket covering the saddle. The dust kicks up as their numbers increase. The tribes are gathering.

Soon 400 Indians are packed in the small holding area between the tepee village and the rodeo grounds where they are about to perform, for the third time today, before the gathered cowboys and cowgirls and lovers of the rodeo circuit.

For such a large gathering, the silence is powerful. Occasionally, a baby's cry is heard. There are soft murmurings among the women near the fence. The older men and boys on horseback sit impassively, staring ahead with dull eyes, not seeming to see anything.

They go where directed by the harsh voice over the loudspeaker and stand between three high chain-link fences just outside the rodeo grounds. It will be some time before they perform. But the rodeo is a tightly run show, choreographed to the last detail, and the extras must be ready to go onstage at a moment's notice. So they stand and wait in the heat.

The traditional clothing is from a time when the people were living with nature in the mountains east of this Oregon town; the thick leather pants, skirts, and blouses are not meant for the heat of this summer day. The heavy breastplates and moccasins cling to the skin, preventing it from breathing. Beads of sweat begin to appear on foreheads. Infants start to cry or whine. The men and women stand pressed together or sit on impatient horses, silently looking ahead, dealing with the place and the heat in practiced stoicism. The sun is intense. No cooling breeze comes to that spot.

"Indians! C'mon, Indians. You're on after the clown act. Indians, get ready."

The cracking voice comes out of nowhere through a loud-speaker above the chain-link fence. No one is visible behind the words. It's a disembodied voice directing the characters in this bizarre theater. The Indians hear but pay little attention.

They simply wait in the sun. They have done this before.

The bull-riding competition has finally ended, and clowns are now rushing about the massive arena, entertaining the full grandstand with slapstick antics. The announcer's voice booms over the sound system with a banter of straight lines to the clowns' sight gags. The crowd is responding well—they have paid to see a good show, and a good show it is. The clowns finish off their act with one last pie in the face and a final exploding jalopy ride around the arena to loud applause and laughter. It's a timeless show, reminiscent of those in the Roman forum on hot Sunday afternoons thousands of years ago. The show has not changed much in all that time.

The crowd checks the program for the next event. Coming up are the "Traditional Indian Dances"—not exactly a highlight, but something entertaining nonetheless. A loud bell rings, signaling the next act. The announcer begins his prepared text.

"Now, ladies and gentlemen, for your pleasure and entertainment, we are extremely proud to present the only Real Americans! Entering the arena at this moment are our great friends, the Indians from the reservation, who will perform for you their ancient social dances. As you can see, they are completely outfitted in colorful costumes, all for your pleasure and entertainment. Aren't they something?"

The spirited monologue continues as the gate between Indian village and arena finally opens. In matching cowboy hats, white shirts, and official badges, two white men at the gate check to make sure everyone is properly ornamented. The people move slowly, silently through the gate.

The air suddenly fills with an unusual sound—quiet, gentle bells worn on leggings and fringed buckskin trousers. It's a powerful and haunting sound, like wind chimes in a gentle breeze. It builds in intensity and rhythm as more people move through the gate and into the dusty arena. The bells compete with the rustle of the crowd. A few people in the grandstand begin to pay attention. Many more file down the aisles to the concession area for another cup of beer, another round of hot dogs.

First come the men and boys on horseback, moving slowly around the periphery toward the large grandstand to the south. Each man raises a feathered handpiece and waves to the crowd, as directed. There are twenty, perhaps thirty prancing horses moving in single file around the arena. Their presence begins to assert itself.

Following the horses through the gate are the people on foot. Hundreds pour slowly onto the grounds. Women and girls. Little children and infants in arms. Young men and boys dressed in war regalia of feathers and beaded breastplates. Young women, dark and beautiful, with long buckskin skirts and single feathers in their black hair, moving onto the rodeo grounds with eyes downcast, not looking at the multitudes in the stands. The only sound is the constant dancing of bells on their moving bodies.

"Our Indian friends will be performing, for your pleasure, some of their ancient dances. Watch the young boys perform the war dance to your left. Watch the women do the circle dance in the center arena. These friends of ours from the reservation have been part of this great show for forty years now, and we welcome them back every year. Aren't they something?"

The people begin to perform without obvious direction. A new sound counters the bells: twelve older men at the rear of the arena begin drumming and chanting around a massive drum. The chant is hypnotic and timeless. It fills the air with infectious pulsations. The people start to dance.

The children are the most active in their movements. They have watched their parents and elders for years and are learning the steps well. Their thin arms and legs jerk out in all directions as they pound the earth with their feet. The drumming and chanting grow louder.

After fifteen minutes, a man in a white cowboy hat and carrying a clipboard swings his arms in front of the stands, letting the dancers know it's time for the rodeo to move on to bareback bronc riding. Indian ceremonial time is up. It doesn't matter whether the dance and song have reached their natural completion—they must stop now, for the next act is waiting.

"Well, folks, that has been the Indian dances for your pleasure and entertainment. The dancers will be back tomorrow, so you can look forward to seeing them again. Our most colorful Americans in the country today—the Real Americans—performing for you today. Let's give them a big hand."

The people filter back through the gate. Their expressions haven't changed. The men on horseback have finished their slow, single circle of the arena and are the first to leave. The dancers follow quietly, bells again providing the only sound except for brief, polite applause from the crowd. The show has come to an end.

At the gate, the same two officials stand on either side, holding large, round rolls of amusement-ride tickets one might find at a county fair. As each Indian passes through the gate, a ticket is torn off and placed in an outstretched hand. A ticket for each person—large or small. After extracting their pay, the people file quietly back to their tepees to take off the ornamental garb and change back into T-shirts, jeans, and cowboy boots. Time to return to normal.

A bottleneck develops at the narrow gate, for the two men cannot keep up with the hundreds of hands reaching for tickets. The now stagnant mass of people spreads out onto the grounds and prevents rodeo workers from setting up barriers for the next riding event. The cowboys ask the people to move off the grounds, forcefully but without pushing. The people press against the gate and chain-link fence. The heat and dust are overwhelming, but they pack together ever more tightly, maintaining their silence. They have been here before. It is useless to protest.

The tickets will later be redeemed for another commodity: money. A dollar or two for every ticket you produce at the end of the rodeo. A few dollars for the dance. The more dances you perform, the more tickets you get to convert into money.

The sun is now lower in the sky, and the rodeo day is coming to a close. Tomorrow will bring the same show, the same heat, the same expectation of tickets at the gate. But for the moment, there is time to sit in front of the tepee and count the tickets and think about the gambling to be done at night. Time for the people to sit and silently look at the sky, and feel the cool earth beneath their legs.

Lost Girl
in the Desert

THE DESERT GETS UNDER ONE'S SKIN without warning. Such a massive expanse of openness and quiet beauty stretches out beyond vision, beyond comprehension of its delicate balance. It is a mystical place, full of new sounds and sights, bringing to memory tales of magic and visions.

The Sonoran Desert of the southwestern United States and northern Mexico spreads over 120,000 square miles in its mystery and beauty. It is pure and unspoiled, with only an occasional scar of civilization seen in pockmarked bombing ranges, gravel mines, and rare settlements. Long arid valleys are suddenly broken by stark, 7,000-foot mountain ranges. Despite a sparse annual rainfall of less than ten inches, vegetation and animal life abound. Cacti, mesquite and paloverde trees, grasses, creosote and salt bushes. All manner of snakes and lizards, small rodents, coyote, javelina, quail, and mule deer.

This is the land of the Tohono O'odham—the Desert People, known also as the Papago. It is the place that has always been their home, the environment they understand and respect. Anthropologists place their residence in the desert at more than 10,000 years, back through the ancestral Hohokam peoples. The O'odham, however, have a different story of their genesis. The original creators, Earth Medicine

Man and I'itoi, gave life to many families of people in the dark time. There were wars and destruction of races. And then I'itoi, the great giver of all things, molded a perfect people and placed them in the desert to grow and prosper. It required a perfect people to survive in that often harsh world. They are the O'odham.

When one looks at the desert in early morning light, there is a perfection of order in its sights, sounds, and smells. It is easy to forget its harshness, its unforgiving character. One forgets that a respect for its power must be constant and diligent. Despite the natural order of all things in the desert, its delicate balance can become violent with the slightest of influences.

I learned much about the desert during those few days she was lost.

DAY ONE

We first received word of her disappearance on a Friday afternoon. I was sitting at my desk in my small cubicle of an office in the tribal health authority building, trying to get through the last hours of a misdirected week. It was midsummer and the days of constant heat and dryness had taken their toll. I could hardly keep my mind on any business, especially something as dry and uninspired as the fourth draft of a community health education plan.

Thoughts kept floating back about how I ended up in that cubicle in the desert heat of July. With the memories came the sadness, as it had so often those past months. I had come to this desert community called Sells on the Tohono O'odham Reservation almost a year before—come with such great hopes and plans. After years of working as a clinical physician with Indian Health Service, I had been strongly recruited to accept the prestigious job as Service Unit Director of the O'odham health system. This was the "model" service unit in the IHS program—a system of hospitals, clinics, doctors and nurses, health educators, and a fleet of vehicles providing health care to the 10,000 O'odham living on a reservation with a land mass greater than the state of Connecticut. It was, for me, the natural culmination of a process to make meaningful changes in how the federal government satisfied its treaty responsibilities to provide cradle-to-grave health care to Indian people.

Joining the O'odham was exciting as well. They were a mysterious and quiet tribe, second only to the Navajo in number, land area, and their tenacious grasp on traditional ways of living and healing. Over the years, I had developed a great respect for traditional Indian practices, and the O'odham appeared to have a unique understanding of how to blend the best from both technological, modern medicine and their traditional ceremonies, medicine people, and herbal remedies. Now I was going to be a part of this bridging of worlds.

I dived into my new administrative role with passion. Long hours and seven-day weeks were common, yet accepted, for there was important work to be done. But then, for reasons still unclear, things began to go wrong.

A few key administrative positions at the hospital went chronically unfilled—forcing me to take on financial management responsibilities for which I had neither the experience nor skills. We were down two physicians and a half-dozen nurses, and everyone was overworked and constantly knocking on my office door with legitimate complaints. One of our public-health nurses had a sudden, intense emotional crisis, decided I was the source of all her problems, and began making threats on my life. I was living alone in the government compound and had little stimulation outside my work. And perhaps most draining to the spirit, the O'odham tribal health board—a very influential group of consumers—found me less an ally than I had hoped. Rather than someone who deeply respected their ways, I was increasingly viewed as just another Anglo bureaucrat insensitive to their needs.

After nine months of mounting frustration and personal anguish, I knew I had to take a different course. I asked the director in Tucson to relieve me of that Service Unit Director's job, to reassign me to something for which I was better suited. We made a mutual arrangement with the tribe to appoint me as medical consultant to the O'odham Health Authority, a collection of innovative community-oriented programs operated by the tribe and under contract with the government.

The relationship had its positive aspects for both me and the authority. But the sense of failure in giving up the director's position remained a wound that was healing too slowly. It was the first major failure I had experienced since being "cut" from the freshman basketball team back in high school, and I was handling the existential crisis poorly. Day after day of sitting in that isolating cubicle further underscored my lack of direction and purpose. The days were long and hot and dry.

We got the call from the tribal police in mid-afternoon. A twenty-year-old mentally retarded girl from the village of Quijotoa was lost in the desert. There had been a family argument, and she had walked away in anger from the little cluster of adobe shacks. She had done this before, since her capacity to speak of her frustrations was forever wanting. When she got mad, she simply ran into the desert—usually for a few hours, occasionally overnight—yet always returned on her own, or was found by her father and uncles.

This time her disappearance was recognized more than two days before, on Tuesday. It wasn't until late Thursday that tribal police had been notified. Her family had attempted a search on their own for two days, as was the custom—to take care of family business in a quiet and nonintrusive way. Now frantic, they had finally contacted the authorities. A minimal search took place late Thursday, but nothing other than a few tracks were found.

Now, on Friday afternoon, a full-scale search was being organized. Someone in the office who heard of it asked if I would go along. Maybe if she was injured, I could help.

I gathered a few medical supplies, two large plastic jugs of water, and a portable two-way radio keyed into the tribal frequency. By late afternoon, I was in my aging four-wheel drive and heading west the twenty-five miles to her village of Quijotoa.

As I traveled alone on that two-lane asphalt highway snaking its way through the desert, the sun was falling toward the western horizon but still baking the land and the inside of my car with its unrelenting heat. Even in the late afternoon the temperature was well over 100 degrees, as it had been almost every day for three months. The summer thunderstorms were beginning to bring occasional relief from the constant pressure of the sun, but most days were like this—clear and scorching hot, with not even a breeze to cool the soul.

My eyes wandered through the expanse of desert surrounding me. Shadows on the mountain ridges were emerging as falling sunlight hit jagged slopes. The forests of stately saguaro cactus, many more than thirty feet tall, covered the sloping hillsides. Each had two to four massive arms reaching toward the heavens, as if a choir of silent worshipers was praying to the sun. Thick creosote bushes had turned brown with the heat. As far as the eye could see, there was nothing but expanse and harsh beauty. No roads, no dwellings, no green lawns of the suburban life just sixty miles to the east, in Tucson. It was beautiful despite the heat.

The hastily called search team was meeting at a rest stop near Quijotoa—called Covered Wells by some—a moderate-size O'odham village of 300 people. As I came over the rise, the widely spaced living compounds of extended families could be seen. Adobe houses were interspersed with more modern prefabricated dwellings recently erected by the tribal housing authority, and with the ever-present outdoor wooden ramadas where much of O'odham life took place during summer months. Meals were prepared under those ocotilla and mesquite tree overhangs. The sleeping cots were outside as well, for the evening coolness of the clear desert air was the only relief from the heat.

I pulled into the rest stop. About a dozen police cars and vans and a few pickups were parked in a row. A collection of men, many in uniform, was standing around a worn picnic bench among the prickly pear and cholla cactus. Off to the side another group—obviously men from the village—stood silently watching the predominantly non-Indian police go over maps spread on a table. Two women at a separate picnic table were tending to pots of coffee and homemade sandwiches. I recognized the uniforms of many jurisdictions: local sheriffs' deputies, state police officers, and tribal police. Although at first I didn't see any familiar faces, I soon spotted Ralph, a friend and fellow health worker who lived in Quijotoa and was assisting with local arrangements. We said hello, and introductions to the various officers were made.

A heavyset, red-faced lieutenant sheriff from the town of Ajo was seemingly in charge. He reported that a set of tracks had already been followed for a few miles from the family house toward the village of Vaya Chin, some twenty miles across the open desert to the northwest. A sister of the lost girl lived in Vaya Chin, and some thought she might be heading in that direction. Despite her mental retardation, the girl was said to be versed in the desert and its landmarks. She could well have known where she was heading.

We learned that some village men were already out on horseback following her footprints in the sandy soil. A few four-wheel drives were also sent out into the open desert as the search became organized. Another base camp was about to be established near a windmill ten miles off the main road, where a secondary search by trackers on foot could be mobilized.

The Anglo police were loud and talkative. They shared laughter and war stories of previous searches, both to find those accidentally lost in the desert and to round up the constant influx of Mexican nationals who came across the border south of there. The O'odham men were standing off by themselves, talking little. I picked up on no sense of real leadership in this search and was uncomfortable with the feeling of a military maneuver. I decided to go to the windmill base camp with Tony, another tribal man I knew, who had just arrived at the rest stop.

Tony and I headed west in my truck, then turned north on a little-used dirt road through the desert. Those barely visible paths through the mesquite and creosote bushes were used infrequently by local villagers as they tended the small herds of wiry cattle that lived off the sparse vegetation. Looking in all directions at the openness, I sensed the enormity of the task. The girl could be almost anywhere. The land was crisscrossed with deep, dry riverbeds called arroyos, which fill only briefly during torrential summer thunderstorms. Small ranges of mountains and hillsides held countless caves and pockets of large rocks that could hide a person from any search party, especially if she didn't want to be found. A few fence lines to keep the cattle in a general area of the desert could be seen in the distance. But most of what Tony and I saw on that ride was a massive, unmanageable openness.

We found no one at the windmill. The radio I had hastily brought along was nonfunctional, so we decided to drive the dusty miles back to the first base camp. There more men and radios were arriving, but a delicate political issue was brewing over who should be in charge—the sheriff or the tribal police. Nothing was resolved, and I grew increasingly uncomfortable with that element of the search.

My four-wheeler was assigned to carry four local men back to the well area so they could continue the search on foot. As we drove through the desert, the heat was still intense and the fine dust raised by my tires filled the back of my rig, causing the men to wheeze and cough. No one complained, however, for it was not the way of these people to fight the desert's reality. "Be silent, be patient, move slowly" were tenets of the O'odham taught since birth.

Our group began a poorly organized track along a series of fence lines near the windmill. I drove slowly, keeping an ear to a borrowed portable radio linked with the base camp and watching the line of searchers on either side of an arroyo. What are we looking for? I wondered. Were her tracks seen in this area? What are the chances that one of us will simply stumble upon her in all this vastness? I radioed the base camp to get direction; they offered none. We called off the tracking and sat near the windmill for more than an hour, waiting for guidance from someone. The men and I talked of simple things, like the heat. An O'odham friend named Pru, with whom I had played basketball in the past, spoke of the upcoming season and what village teams looked tough to beat. We waited and waited as the sun descended on the western horizon and a coolness came to the night air.

In the fading light of dusk, we made one last search for signs of tracks along the fence line. A nice wind came up and evaporated the sweat on our foreheads. The last shadows caught the cactus and rocks, producing the incredible color that the desert displays at sundown. Two files of quiet trackers moved along the lines. All we could hear was the rubbing of salt bush on jeans and the evening calls of birds in the mesquite trees.

With darkness quickly falling, the men in four-wheelers and those on foot regrouped near the windmill. There was an excitement in the air, for despite the lack of results, our search now seemed better organized. Tony and I sat on the hood of my truck watching the trackers coming in over the hillsides. Two distinct groups were gathering. The predominantly non-Indian officers with their CB radios and guns on hips were talking incessantly, chain-smoking cigarettes. Off to the side, the local men from surrounding villages were saying little, yet communicating extensively with facial and hand gestures. As I watched them, they seemed intently serious about this business. They knew the desert, especially its often harsh and unforgiving side. And the girl was one of their own. She was young and afraid and lost in the desert. I could see the look of great concern on their faces.

We finally returned in darkness to the rest area near Quijotoa. Moving through the desert, the lights of my truck caught glimpses of night animals scurrying across the landscape. Shadows jumped into consciousness, then disappeared. Bizarre shapes of cactus and scrub bushes flickered across the eyes. I felt like I was traveling through a foreign place—through the Australian outback or a dreamscape of my own mind.

It was ten o'clock by the time we arrived. Harsh floodlights from a dozen police cars illuminated the picnic tables, where sandwiches and coffee were again being served. Plans were made for the search to continue by first light. Again the various players were in competition for command—the sheriff's group, tribal police, and now even more men, including Bureau of Indian Affairs officers, tribal government leaders, and local village headmen. But everyone was too tired for arguments, and the meeting broke up quickly.

I drove back to my trailer in Sells, where sleep came quickly and easily.

Day Two

My harsh alarm clock was buzzing for minutes before it raised my consciousness. My throat felt on fire from the dust and heat of the previous evening's search. It was Saturday—a day to sleep in—but I forced myself up, washed quickly, grabbed a few supplies, and was heading west again by 5:45 A.M.

First light of the desert morning was glowing above the tall mountains to the east. The sweet smell of morning freshness filled my dusty truck and a coolness was in the air, for rain had fallen briefly while we slept. I could hear morning birds calling loudly across the desert; flickers and flycatchers were out on their early rounds. An occasional hoot could be heard from an owl returning from its nightly hunt. The nocturnal animals were slipping back into their burrows, and the few creatures tolerant of the summer sun were beginning to move about. The cycle of a new day in that beautiful, balanced place was beginning.

The search group was regathering at the rest stop as I pulled in. More police types were present. A few horseback riders from the village were already out in search of the girl's tracks from the day before. Initial word coming to the base camp was that her tracks had been found farther toward the Vaya Chin area. So a decision was made to set up a new camp in that village and expand the search from both directions.

The brief thunderstorm that had swept through in the night was not forceful enough to destroy most tracks, so there was optimism. Some lingering clouds remained to the northwest. This day would be cooler, the sun less oppressive.

There was a long discussion at the rest stop on the best way to regroup at Vaya Chin—either by the paved road, which was a long trip of almost sixty miles, or overland across the desert, a distance of twenty miles with the possibility of washed-out arroyos and impassable dirt roads.

I headed out overland on my own, with a false sense of security that my four-wheeler could surmount anything. The rain had lessened the dust, and the trip into the desert was cool and stimulating. I reached another windmill area, which had been designated as the meeting spot for trackers and horse riders already out. Our radio system was faring better than the previous day as we gathered to begin the search from that point.

The riders reported that new tracks had been found where the girl had gone under a fence line about a mile from our location. Her father and two brothers were already in that area on foot, continuing the search on their own. I thought of them walking alone in the desert, catching an occasional glimpse of a track, a broken branch where their little girl had stumbled. It was now almost four days since her disappearance. I couldn't conceive of the agony felt during their grim and endless search.

By mid-morning the clouds were breaking and heat was again coming to the desert. Because of the brief rains, a heaviness of unusual humidity was in the air. I had elected to stay with the trackers as the source of radio contact rather than go with the sheriff to the new base camp in Vaya Chin.

We were walking along a fence line, looking for tracks, when we saw a group of large turkey vultures circling above a cluster of thick mesquite trees up ahead. Scavengers of the desert, the vultures were part of the cycle of life and death—everything was returned to the natural chain in one form or another. It was a sure sign that death had occurred up ahead. We hastened our pace toward that group of trees, fearing what we might find. Within fifty yards of the spot, the unmistakable smell of rotting flesh struck us. Two young men ran ahead, then returned quickly to report it was the decaying carcass of a cow, a familiar sight during summer months when the rare rainfall and sparse vegetation made life so fragile for those thin and mournful beasts. I reflected on the lost girl's fragility, as well. The desert makes no distinction between humans and cows when its unrelenting heat withers the body.

We kept walking through the morning hours. The uneven terrain and hidden rocks caused my ankles to twist suddenly. My legs and back became stiff and fatigued. Despite my thick jeans and heavy boots, the sharp spines of cholla cactus and salt bush scraped my ankles and thighs. We walked and walked, yet the enormity of the place was overwhelming. The search seemed endless, the quest impossible.

Far out in the desert, the trackers and I rendezvoused at a *charco*, a manmade earthen water tank shaped when a bulldozer had raised four dirt walls to form a ten-foot-long rectangle that would collect the summer rains for thirsty cattle. There I learned by radio that aircraft were now helping with the search. We set up a small base camp. Soon searchers on foot and horseback wandered in from the desert to join us. There was stillness, then a flurry of motion as six men arrived, then stillness again until the next group came. The *charco* became a magnet, drawing everyone together.

We sat on the lip of the *charco* and talked quietly. The promise of a cooler day had now evaporated like the water in the bone-dry walls under our hips. The heat was growing in intensity. Pesky flies buzzed at our faces, our necks. We drank water from plastic jugs, but it was already hot and did little to moisten our parched throats.

We received a sudden radio call that the horsemen had found new tracks, pointed eastward. The lost girl had abruptly changed course, almost 120 degrees from her original path. After so many miles of walking northwest toward Vaya Chin, she had turned and was heading east toward a larger settlement called Santa Rosa.

Why did she turn? Did she suddenly want to go home and instead get confused while retracing her steps? Was she disoriented from heat and dehydration? Many thoughts poured through me. She had been so close to a small village near Vaya Chin, but in turning east she was now again in open, vast desert. The nearest village or road was thirty miles away.

I decided to take some trackers back to Vaya Chin and regroup there. The horsemen were still following her tracks toward the east. I radioed them and set up another rendezvous for later that afternoon. The US Border Patrol—self-styled experts in desert searches—had joined the fray and were approaching her possible position from the Santa Rosa area. In addition, a military helicopter had been searching near the horsemen. Activity was at a peak.

The base camp at Vaya Chin was under a large ramada by the old elementary school. Finally, we got a bit of shade and soda pop as we sat under the trees. The sense of a military maneuver again prevailed—maps laid out on the tables, radios buzzing, men talking loudly and smoking cigarettes.

The teams of searchers were fed leather-hard hamburgers and slightly warm pop in the school cafeteria. As I stood in line to get my plate, I watched the two teenage Indian girls serving food. One was very pretty and thin, perhaps about fifteen years old. Perfect dark skin and shining white teeth. She seemed a goddess of the desert—shy, mysterious, timeless. Her life was ahead of her, and possibilities limitless.

I thought of the lost girl. Twenty years old, mentally retarded, forever frustrated, and locked into an existence for which she was not responsible. And now she was alone and afraid in that vastness. Two separate women of the desert—different chances in life, different journeys taken.

Plans were made for a new base camp in Santa Rosa, about thirty miles due east. I spoke privately with a tribal police captain who, having become increasingly frustrated with the sheriff's leadership, had decided to take eight men on his own to search a deserted O'odham village south of Santa Rosa, on the chance she may have wandered there. The O'odham traditionally lived in summer and winter homes on a regular cycle changing with the seasons. Winters were spent in the arid valleys, while in summers families would relocate to the mountains, hunting game and escaping the killer heat. The captain knew of such a winter settlement; and having visited it once myself, I arranged to bring food and water to his men there later in the day.

Just as I was leaving with a group of men to begin a search in the vicinity of Santa Rosa, I was commandeered by the sheriff in charge to take him to establish a new base near that community. I felt like protesting, but found it impossible to refuse. Like him, I was an official Anglo officer. But I would much rather have been on foot or horseback with the local trackers.

I drove the lieutenant sheriff and another officer along the main

road between Vaya Chin and Santa Rosa. All the while, I kept looking to my right, to the open desert to the south. She must be in that
area, I thought. The tracks can't be wrong.

A welcome afternoon thunderstorm was forming over the desert,
and we could feel a breeze rising in the west. But there was no rain yet,
and wind brought only more stifling heat and the ever-present dust.

We turned off the main road near a cemetery south of Santa
Rosa and headed due west into the desert. Using our radios, we rendezvoused with several searchers on horseback and in four-wheelers.
The Border Patrol (BP) was there in full force now—three tan vehicles
designed for desert travel and a dozen uniformed men with large guns
on their hips. The BP officers were anxious to join in, excited about
the "hunt," as they called it. They made me nervous as they roared
across the desert, roiling up the dust.

The radio brought word that fresh tracks had been found in an
arroyo about half a mile from our location. It seemed they were those
of the lost girl—and to our surprise, a dog was with her. She has a
companion, I thought. She is lost, but perhaps not alone. A friend is
with her, and one better equipped for survival than she.

Everyone sensed we were near her. She was close.

We traveled overland to the arroyo with fresh tracks. I bent down
and looked carefully. Yes—there were the tracks of simple leather-
soled sandals, and to one side, the paw prints of a dog. I watched a
policeman take snapshots and measurements of the prints as though
it were a crime scene. Some trackers on foot were following the trail
over the hillsides toward the west. Expectations were high. The helicopter landed nearby, kicking up a breath-stopping cloud of dust.

Suddenly, one of the local searchers made a choking sound deep
in his throat and fell to the ground in a grand mal epileptic seizure—
not an uncommon occurrence on a reservation replete with heavy
drinking and with head injuries from earlier wild days. I instinctively
became a doctor again as I gave the man an injection to stop the con-
vulsion. I tried to persuade the helicopter pilot to transport him back
to the hospital in Sells, but the young flier was reluctant. He didn't

want to miss the triumph now that we seemed so close.

I stayed with the semiconscious man to make sure he was stable. The seizures had stopped; he had suffered no other injuries. It was strange but comforting to be the doctor again. I had not been touching patients for almost a year now, because the administrative job had allowed very little time in the clinic. An old, friendly feeling was coming into my life again as I rechecked the man's blood pressure.

Rapid communications began crackling on the radios. Underwear had been found hanging on a tree branch just over the rise in front of us. The off-white panties were brought back in a sealed plastic bag and given to the lieutenant. He examined them closely and commented on "secretions around the crotch area." I winced.

A few moments passed. Finally, a radio message came through from the Border Patrol team. Excitement grabbed us all as we strained to listen for details.

"She's been found—they have the girl." Then three seconds later: "She's dead." The radio went silent.

A stillness fell over the group. No one said a word. Then a flurry of activity—calls to the base camps in Vaya Chin and Santa Rosa, radio relays to horsemen and trackers on foot, to end the search. It was all very official.

I had two competing feelings, both intense. One was a sense of loss, for the girl was dead. She had become a part of me and everyone else on that search. Yet I also felt exhilaration and relief. It had been a long journey, physically and spiritually painful. I was relieved it was over, that the search had achieved some measure of success, however sad.

The Indians in the group were quiet, busying themselves by gathering gear and straightening up the camp. The non-Indians were more vocal and seemed happy with the discovery, the closure. Some backslapping and congratulations went on.

The helicopter took to the skies to mark the spot for others coming in. I offered to officially pronounce her dead, in keeping with my role there, although I felt strange about my need to be so official and medical at such a time and place. My offer was accepted by the sheriff.

We traveled in four-wheelers over a few hills to the west. What could barely pass for a road suddenly stopped, however, and we had to go on foot about 200 yards over another rise.

It was a strange sight. Two Border Patrol vehicles were parked off to the right. On the left was a group of seven O'odham on horseback. All were silent, staring toward a solitary paloverde tree on a slight rise. I couldn't see the body. No one was speaking.

Dark clouds from a gathering thunderstorm now covered the sky. I felt frightened by the silence and the clouds. It was almost as if I were in a church of strange denomination, unsure of what ceremony was to be performed.

Three of us walked silently up the rise toward the paloverde— me, the lieutenant, and an O'odham officer. We stepped in each others' footprints so as not to disturb other marks. As we neared the tree, her body became obvious. She was lying rigid, partially erect against its trunk. Her arms and legs appeared bloated and were jutting out in an unnatural, grotesque way. A simple white handkerchief, stained with sweat, had been placed over her face by whoever had been first on the scene.

I approached. It was a simple picture: the paloverde tree with its small brownish leaves; her body resting against the rough bark of its trunk. A small red transistor radio attached to a round chain lay to the right of her head. On the left, almost within arm's reach, lay an empty glass jar on its side, its screw top close by. It was her jar of water, long since empty, unable to provide her with any relief from the desert's heat and dryness. I wondered: How long had she been carrying that jar since its last drops were gulped? How long did she cling to it after her lips were parched and her mind was hallucinating from the heat?

We decided not to disturb anything until the Bureau of Indian Affairs (BIA) deputy arrived. I approached the Indian horsemen and exchanged a few words. Mainly, we stood in silence.

The helicopter came back with the BIA policeman. He was well dressed in tailored pants, new boots, and a string tie. He carried a clipboard, a camera, and a white plastic body-bag. He and I walked up to the body. He began the meticulous process of taking pictures and collecting evidence to be placed in sealed bags.

I removed the cloth from her face. Some decomposing had already taken place, for her eyes were sunken and opaque. Flies and ants were busy around her eyes and mouth. Dirt covered her lips and teeth. I thought she was probably pretty in life—slightly bucked teeth, but a nice face. I could imagine her playing and laughing around the family home in Quijotoa.

From the condition of the body, she must have already been dead a few days. She might even have settled down by the tree, exhausted and dehydrated, before we embarked on our search—on those long days of walking, tracking, looking for footprints to lead the way. No tracks were fresh, no leads promising. It had been a quest without a goal. It had been needless wandering.

As we prepared to place her in the body bag, the groups of horsemen, police, and four-wheel drivers slowly broke up and headed back toward their respective villages and towns. I stayed a while, helping load her into a Border Patrol van for transport to Tucson and the autopsy.

I drove back to Santa Rosa with two young Indians from the search. We spoke little, except while stopping to help another four-wheel vehicle out of a rain-filled gully. Rains had finally come to the earth again. The air was cool and sweet with freshness. A low sun broke beneath the clouds to the west, giving magical colors and contrasts to the desert. The evening seemed quiet and peaceful. There was a sense of ending.

We reached Santa Rosa by dark. Many people from the village were gathered with those involved in the search. We exchanged some quiet talk and shared chile, beans, and hamburgers. I wasn't hungry, but politely accepted the food.

I went back to Quijotoa to meet with the family. A small crowd had gathered at their place, giving them support and sharing their pain. There were few tears, for most had already feared the worst. I made some embarrassing apologies.

Finally alone on my drive back to Sells, I let my thoughts wander. I reflected on our journeys—the potentially fatal wanderings all of us take in life. Because of an argument or misunderstanding, we head off in a new direction into uncharted, sometimes hostile lands. We feel lost. We are afraid, yet can't seem to go back. We get confused and turned around. Everything gets turned around.

Will someone come searching for us when we're lost? Will they find us in time?

Feeling numb, I continued on through the evening desert coolness. Back at the trailer, I hastily called the woman in Tucson I was to see that evening and made brief apologies. I fixed a stiff drink and sat in the darkness, reflecting again. I had to make decisions. It was time to figure out where I was going. Tomorrow I would begin that process.

At last, I fell into a restless sleep. Dreams of the desert kept coming. Dreams of the beauty and the balance and the heat.

Walk into Baboquivari

IN THE BEGINNING THERE WAS NOTHING but darkness, and the earth was not finished. There was water and blackness and lapping sounds, as in a pond. Then a strong wind blew, and First Born came into the darkness. He was cold and alone. He prayed to Earth Medicine Man and was told how to finish the earth and how to make light in the sun and moon and stars. After he had prepared the earth and sky, First Born went away.

The sky came down and met the earth, and the first one to come forth was I'itoi, Elder Brother. Earth Medicine Man and I'itoi became busy making races of people to inhabit the earth. But then there were wars and floods. Many races were destroyed. Earth Medicine Man and I'itoi battled, whereupon Earth Medicine Man disappeared, leaving the world to his opponent. I'itoi then created a new race, strong and giving, and put them in a place where only a special people could survive. I'itoi drove away the previous inhabitants, who fled eastward and became the Apache. The new people flourished in that special place, the desert. They were called the Tohono O'odham—the Desert People.

After the work was done, I'itoi returned to his home in the center of the world, on a mountain peak called Baboquivari. There he remains to this day. I'itoi can be heard singing as he sits on his woven mat, grinding his cornmeal on a metate. His song is the wind coming down from Baboquivari—the sacred place, home of I'itoi, Elder Brother.

The sun rises in the east over Baboquivari each new morning in that land. The sharp, barren summit of Baboquivari catches the last light of dusk. This peak dominates the expanse of the Tohono O'odham desert land, and can be seen from virtually every point in the four sacred directions. It is the center, the place of the Creator.

The Tohono O'odham still live in that place, which I'itoi chose for them. And Baboquivari is still there, dominating both their landscape and their spirituality. Their prayers are sent to the mountain— prayers for the healing, for the rain, for the birth of a new one into their family. Medicine people make a journey to Baboquivari at special times to gather the sacred plants and rocks that contain the Power. Individual O'odham travel to Baboquivari on private journeys of awareness and vision. It is the magnet for much of their lives.

Baboquivari looks like a magnet. It stands stark and alone in the midst of the Sonoran Desert of the southwestern United States and northern Mexico. The Sonoran Desert sprawls across 120,000 square miles and consists of long, arid valleys interspersed with mountain ranges of treeless, rocky peaks. Baboquivari is the highest point in that desert, standing majestically at 7,730 feet. It is an almost perfectly shaped cone of granite, bare and brighter in color than the surrounding mountain range. When the evening light catches its apex long after the sun has disappeared behind the western horizon, Baboquivari beams with an incredible glow. It is a fitting home for I'itoi, creator of O'odham.

I had been living in the land of O'odham for a year. My home was in the town of Sells, capital of the Tohono O'odham Nation, sixty-five miles west of Tucson. My arrival was full of excitement and promise. I had accepted a job as director of the government-operated health system for the 10,000 O'odham tribal members living on the reservation. It seemed the natural culmination of my career with Indian Health Service, for I had been moving steadily from being a practicing physician at small clinics in isolated reservation settings to becoming an administrator of hospitals and health programs.

The O'odham health system was unique in a number of ways. It was the IHS "model" service unit, with strong input from its Office of Research and Development in Tucson, which was forever coming up with new techniques and procedures for improving health care among Indian people. And the O'odham tribe itself had established a powerful health authority, which not only operated its own community health services under contract with the government but also took a strong role in overseeing the IHS system of hospitals, clinics, physicians, nurses, and technicians.

My stint as Service Unit Director at Sells was short-lived and undistinguished. Despite my enthusiasm and what I thought were skills for bridging the worlds of technological and traditional medicine, things had not gone well. Some miscalculations here, a string of bad-luck occurrences there, and simply being caught in a slippery slide of no-win situations all together made my nine months as director a progressively draining experience.

I asked to be transferred from the position. A mutually agreeable compromise was arranged where I became the medical consultant to O'odham tribal health services under a government assignment. Working directly with the tribe and its perspective on health care had a freshness to it. No longer was I tied down to mundane bureaucratic details. I was free to spend most days talking with local village groups, tribal committees, and traditional Indian healers. There was laughter instead of grumbling. Optimism instead of reliving failures of the past. And time to reflect on what had brought me to that place.

Despite the positive changes, it was not a pleasant time for me. The sense of failure was a constant companion. I was living in the hospital compound, in a small, roach-infested trailer instead of the spacious and luxurious director's house I had once occupied. I had isolated myself from the non-Indian physicians, nurses, and their families living nearby. Although I had a few O'odham friends, my social life was transient and unfulfilling.

And the season was summer. Summer in the desert with unrelenting day after day of temperatures in the 100s, the constant weight
of sun without the relief of rain, and dust-filled air from afternoon
windstorms.

I felt undirected and lost, like a small dinghy with neither rudder
nor charts.

Was I supposed to be a physician, to return to clinical practice
that had become all too frustrating? I had concluded that much of
"Western" medicine was geared toward simply subduing symptoms
rather than dealing with the real basis of illness—namely, the disharmony
of body, spirit, and the environment. Was I to continue as a commissioned officer with Indian Health Service, to take each new assignment as it appeared and finish off my twenty years of service in a small
cubicle at IHS headquarters in Rockville, Maryland? Was I to continue
my journey toward working directly with tribes such as the O'odham,
to assist them in regaining control over their own health destiny?

With the lack of direction, I also felt the acute loss of a spirituality. I had been raised in an Irish Catholic setting, where the church
was a cornerstone. Although I didn't go to Catholic schools (my non-
denominational father wouldn't tolerate that), I was a devout Catholic
youngster, and served as an altar boy even through college. But then
things changed. For a variety of reasons, I lost the faith, dropped from
the church, and totally rejected not only the teachings of Catholicism
but any trust that there was a single, omnipotent deity at all. My spirituality became that of the present, the individual human soul, and
humankind's collective fight against oppression. There were no longer
heavens and hells. Existentialism became my banner. God was dead.

That creed had led me through medical school and my early
days as a physician. It had, I thought, served me well. But as the centers
of my world began melting like a block of ice in that summer heat, the
lack of a spiritual base left me feeling more alone, more undirected.

One evening I was sitting on the rickety wooden steps leading
up to my trailer, watching the sunset, and yearning for a whiff of breeze
to cut the stifling heat. Looking toward the southeast, I centered on the

distant peak of Baboquivari, brightly lit by the faraway sun, standing stark and solitary above the desert. I had learned from my O'odham friends that Baboquivari held a special place in their culture and religion. I knew of some who spoke of the journeys they took there—journeys for prayers and visions, for answers to important questions in their lives. Baboquivari was reportedly the place where their creator lived. Its spirituality was well-known.

Over the years of living with Indian people in Arizona, New Mexico, and Oregon, I had come to learn and respect many of the traditional Indian ways. Each tribe has its unique mythology of creation and relationship to the universe, yet all groups have similarities in their spiritual base. Most believe in the concept of the Great Spirit. There is a reverence for the entities Mother Earth and Father Sky. Most groups recognize that a spirit exists in all things—people, rocks, plants, animals, the air, the wind—and that these essences are interconnected and dependent upon one another. And all believe that whereas illness comes to humankind when disharmony develops, healing requires restoring the balance between body, spirit, and the world outside.

That pantheistic view of the universe had become my new spirituality over those years. It wasn't well practiced all the time, but I did find comfort and strength in the elements of nature: the mountains and deserts, animals of the earth, the sky, the wind. The outdoors had become my church, the sounds of animals my choir.

I thought of such matters as I watched Baboquivari. It was then I decided that I must take a walk into Baboquivari. I desperately needed the strength that spirituality can offer the human experience, and perhaps walking into the home of I'itoi was the way to find it.

Cautiously and with some embarrassment, I began asking subtle questions of coworkers at the tribal health authority. Was there a certain route one should take into the mountain? Was there some ritual to be performed? Most of my naive questions were greeted with either laughter or a turned back. Such matters were not talked about.

Then one night, Faithe came to my trailer. Faithe was an O'odham woman in her late twenties who worked for the tribal mental health group. Although she spent most of her time in Tucson helping teenage Indians face the difficulties of urban life, we had worked together on a few projects over the previous year and had developed a cautious yet warm relationship.

"I hear you want a vision," Faithe said, a wide grin on her round face and laughter in her voice. It was good to laugh at such things, for I was taking all of this much too seriously.

"Well," she added, "I have no recipe for you, but if you must go, here is something that may help on the journey."

Faithe reached into the canvas bag slung over her shoulder and produced a handmade dark leather pouch with many long fringes hanging from its lower end. In the center of the oblong pouch was a design of blue, yellow, and green beads. And in three places, equidistant around the beadwork, were very old, slightly tarnished, round medallions of Indian silverwork.

I cautiously took the pouch from her. It was soft in my hands. A sweet smell of fresh herbs reached my nose. I found myself lost for words, but as I tried to thank her, she brushed off any further discussion of the pouch and turned our conversation to other matters. We had a few beers, listened to music, and talked easily of mutual friends in Tucson.

After Faithe left, I loosened the light-colored leather thong at the pouch's top. Inside were three small bundles of tan leather, each fashioned into a little bag. Slowly, I opened the tiny pouches.

In the smallest was an off-yellow powder that appeared to be cornmeal. In another bundle was what I recognized as leaves of dried blue sage. And in the third were small pebbles of many colors.

I decided to walk into Baboquivari the following morning. The day, like most over the previous three months, began already hot and grew in intensity as the sun rose higher in the sky. I gathered a few provisions in a small daypack: a plastic canteen of water, fruit, matches, a knife, binoculars, and the dark leather medicine bag Faithe had given me.

Ten miles south of Sells, just beyond the small village of Topowa,

I turned off the main highway onto the long, dusty dirt road leading east toward Baboquivari. I had been on that road before, having made a few trips to the campground at Baboquivari's base for day-hikes and picnics with friends. Today would be a journey without friends, however.

The desert was beautiful in the morning light. The ribbon of a dirt road wound over slightly rolling foothills and through dry arroyos. Far in the distance, Baboquivari stood solitary and dark. Tall saguaro cactus, hundreds of years old, flanked either side of the road like stately, ridged columns. Creosote bushes, scrub mesquite trees, and an occasional paloverde tree covered the dry expanse. My four-wheel-drive Blazer kicked up plumes of fine dust as it bounced down the irregular road.

I had been spending more and more time in the desert since leaving the director's position a few months earlier. It had become a part of the healing process. I was learning more about the plants and animals of the region. I saw Gila woodpeckers, gilded flickers, and screech owls making their nests in small, carved-out depressions in the cool interior of saguaros. I became aware of where rattlesnakes sun themselves to regain warmth after the cool desert nights, and of how to avoid inadvertently stepping into their world. I experienced the sudden fear of being caught in a dry, high-walled arroyo where a torrent of water can appear without warning from thunderstorms miles away. And becoming lost in the desert, I learned, can be frightening, sometimes fatal, even to those who respect its harsh balances.

Because the ten-mile dirt road took almost an hour to navigate, I arrived at the small picnic ground at Baboquivari's base by mid-morning. No other cars were there, which did not surprise me, for people seldom came to this place on a weekday. I was thankful for the promised solitude.

I sat on a deserted picnic table for some time before setting off up the mountain. That little picnic ground was in disrepair, and litter could be seen in the gullies and behind rocks. Between the tables stood tall cottonwood trees, many of which had been critically scarred with etchings and carved messages from thousands of visitors' penknives. Why do they leave their marks on nature? I wondered.

From that point at the base of Baboquivari, the peak was not visible. I knew it was to the north, but the foothills hid much of the mountain's upper reaches. I could see the trail before me. It was time to begin the journey.

The trail up Baboquivari was well traveled, for it was considered a nice day-hike for people in Tucson seeking escape from the oppressive heat of late spring and summer. The lower two miles were an easy walk, a family affair on a lazy Sunday outing. But few hikers passed the halfway point, where the trail got much steeper and required the skills and stamina of technical rock climbers.

For serious climbers the trek to the summit was little more than a mild workout—nothing like the 5.6 difficulty of Yosemite's sheer cliffs. And waiting for them at the top was a sign-in book, placed there by a mountaineering club, to document the many who made it all the way. I had been told the book was already into its second volume.

Months before, I had almost reached the summit with a group of doctors from the Indian hospital. We had attacked the mountain in a macho fashion, poorly equipped and inexperienced in established rock-climbing techniques. We became stymied at a point where a relatively sheer cliff blocked our way, and we had none of the proper ropes, carabiners, or chocks to scale it. So we walked back down, each one of us secretly thankful that we didn't have to face the even more difficult final ascent.

But getting to the summit was not my purpose this time. I'itoi would not be at the summit—that would be too easy and predictable. The gods don't work that way, I mused. I'itoi wouldn't be caught dead surrounded by tourists with cameras and sign-in books. No, my journey that day would take a different route.

Unfortunately, I had no idea where I was going. My walk into Baboquivari needed to just happen, not be planned in great detail. I wanted simply to walk with the mountain and let whatever guide I had within me lead the way.

I hiked up the lower trail with ease. It was wide and well worn, with few rocks to trip up my hurried pace. The trail wound gradually up the mountainside through groves of scrub oak, piñon, pine, and an occasional cottonwood tree. Although the morning was growing hot, my mood was upbeat.

After an hour, the trees began disappearing and the trail grew steeper. No visible walkway remained. I simply had to proceed along the rocky plateaus and inclines of dark-colored boulders in the general direction of northeast.

Up and up I went, the route growing ever less established and more difficult. I was suddenly facing a steep incline of smooth rock, fifty degrees in angle, with no way around to either the right or left. I felt a chill of fear, for the incline had few handholds and one slip could mean a fall of more than 100 feet into a rocky canyon below. I should have told someone I was going up the mountain, I thought. A fall could be fatal, for even if the drop didn't kill me, I could be there for days before anyone would think to mount a search. But this was to be a private journey, and revealing my plans would have diluted the purpose.

I slowly, carefully scaled the steep incline and came across another easy stretch of climbing. From there, for the first time, I could see Baboquivari's summit, above and to the left of me. It was craggy and treeless. From my vantage point, there seemed no obvious route along its stark rock face. The air was growing cooler at that altitude, and I could sense afternoon clouds forming over the peak. A breeze kicked up, causing me to shiver through my T-shirt, now damp with sweat. I walked on, trying to ignore the sudden temperature change.

Soon I came to another sheer face of rock, perhaps fifty feet high. At various points on the wall, climbers had left pitons embedded in cracks, and a nylon rope stretched between the metal anchors leading toward the summit. I bypassed that route upward and chose instead a slow, difficult climb over large boulders the size of trucks. My legs ached as I pushed on. I had broken from the traditional trail to the top, and had no idea where this new path would lead.

The air was much colder now and dark, angry clouds filled the sky in all directions. My hands were bleeding from small cuts and scrapes. My shins burned and my shoulders began cramping. Increasingly, I felt lost. And alone.

Pausing briefly to catch my breath, I reflected on this painful journey. What was I trying to prove? Did I expect this O'odham god to suddenly pop out from behind a boulder, pat me on the shoulder, and say, "There, there, everything is going to be all right"? I no longer had a sense of purpose in my walk. I was frightened, cold, and lost.

I kept moving on, over large rocks, for another hour. Finally, I reached an open, flat area about the size of a living room. Sheer walls rose on three sides of the plateau, and a massive rock overhang stood to my right, forming a natural cavelike depression. There appeared no way around it—only straight up one of the vertical walls. Thunder from a growing storm clapped and echoed against the canyons of stone. A cold and stiff wind whistled angrily through the stone.

I began to cry. Spontaneous sobs racked my body as the sadness and anger of months passed through me. Cold, trapped, and unable to go on, all I could do was release my tears.

I decided to offer prayers to Elder Brother right where I was. No cosmic sign or inner sense told me this was the place; I simply could go no farther.

I reached into my daypack and brought forth the medicine pouch. What was I supposed to do? Was there a way to use the medicine? Perhaps the way was within me.

I knelt on the cold plateau and arranged baseball-size rocks in a circular pattern. I opened one of the small leather bags and arranged the dried sage within the circle of rocks. I had heard that burning sage was part of many healing events, although I had never experienced it directly. As I tried to light the sage with safety matches, the cold wind whipping across the ground extinguished each flame within seconds. Finally, with some patience, I got the sage to begin smoldering. Its dark blue smoke gave off a rich aroma.

I opened the smallest bag and sprinkled cornmeal on the burning sage. It crackled and hissed as the smoke rose in that solitary place.

What prayers was I supposed to say? My mind raced. I had not officially prayed in fifteen years. What words could possibly come after such a long time?

My head spun. My lips could not move. My mind flashed on the incense-laden air and brightly colored vestments of priests.

Heavenly Father, I am truly sorry for having offended Thee . . .

Bless me, Father, for I have sinned . . .

Hail Mary, full of grace . . .

Mea culpa, mea culpa, mea maxima culpa . . .

My thoughts flew to Indian songs. Sing, sing the prayers. What words? I don't know the songs; they are not my songs . . .

A deep, guttural moan arose from within my chest. I forced my voice to give forth a harsh song: "Yeh . . . ha yeh . . . ha ha yeh . . ."

Squatting on the ground, my arms wrapped tightly around my chest and shoulders, I shivered and rocked myself like an infant, sending out a made-up song of prayer, breathing in the acrid dark smoke of sage and blue corn. I then began crying again—deep, purging sobs.

I opened the final pouch of multicolored stones. Rolling them in my hands for a long time, I tried to feel whatever power they could transmit. Finally, I spontaneously threw the stones far off into the granite canyons below and watched them disappear from view.

I know not how long I was in that place. Eventually, I realized the sage had become a charred mass in the center of the stones, and my tears could no longer come.

The wind seemed less cold and biting. Instead of screaming sounds around the rocks, a comforting silence settled on that spot. My shivering stopped.

I had had no visions. I had heard no voices nor seen the way home. There had been no sudden transformation or insight. I felt little, except for a draining of the pain in my shoulders and legs.

I began the long walk back down the mountain. I felt disappointed in the journey and a bit embarrassed about my made-up songs and rituals. The walk down, however, was quick and easy. My pace soon became smoother, and the bounce returned to my steps. The threatening storm had not materialized. In fact, the sun broke through the low clouds to the west, bringing warmth and comfort to my body.

By early evening I was again sitting on a picnic table at the campground, devouring the fruit I had left untouched on the long trip upward. The drive back to Sells, through the wonderful colors and contrasts of evening in the desert, passed without much thought. I let my eyes wander over the rolling expanse and the sunset of yellow, red, orange, and purple.

I never spoke to anyone of that journey to Baboquivari. Faithe and I saw each other often over the next several weeks, but we did not mention the medicine pouch. I worked for another three months with the O'odham health authority and felt positive about what we did for each other. Come fall, I moved back to Santa Fe to begin a new chapter of my life and to rejoin old friends long missed over the miles between us.

Yet each day before my departure from the land of O'odham, I would find myself gazing at Baboquivari standing solitary and glowing in the evening light. With my eyes fixed on the home of I'itoi, I would catch myself smiling.

The Power and
Balance of Healing

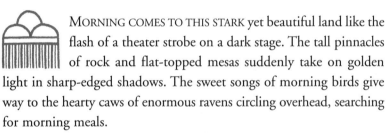MORNING COMES TO THIS STARK yet beautiful land like the flash of a theater strobe on a dark stage. The tall pinnacles of rock and flat-topped mesas suddenly take on golden light in sharp-edged shadows. The sweet songs of morning birds give way to the hearty caws of enormous ravens circling overhead, searching for morning meals.

The deep blue sky seems so close it can almost be touched. Standing alone in the high desert of the Southwest in the crisp morning, one feels power, solitude, and harmony. The land speaks of these qualities. And the people of this land, who lived here centuries before European explorers thought they had discovered an uninhabited paradise, share with it a similar power and a quiet awareness of the way things fit together.

I came to this land and began living with these people in the early 1970s. After four years at Bucknell University and four more intense ones at the University of Pennsylvania, I joined the US Public Health Service and was assigned to one of its branches, Indian Health Service in Arizona. Although most of my medical school colleagues were set in residency programs and nicely aligned to establish themselves on the East Coast, I longed to get away from the noise, bustle, and frenetic pace of the megatropolis. Of equal importance, I was searching desperately for a way to avoid participating in a war I vehemently opposed, and Indian Health Service was a humane alternative that seemed to satisfy my needs.

So my wife and I packed all our belongings into a Dodge van and, along with our street mutt Phredde, traveled across the wondrous expanse of this country and arrived at my duty station—a timeless place called Peach Springs, Arizona.

Peach Springs is the capital, population center, and trading area for the Hualapai Indian Nation, a little-known band of 3,000 people who live on a million-acre reservation along the South Rim of the Grand Canyon in northern Arizona. I was there to run a small four-room clinic, providing all the "Western" health care the Hualapai people would have available. Additionally, once every two weeks I was to ride by horseback down a nine-mile rugged switchback trail into the Canyon to visit with the Havasupai, a unique tribe of 430 who live in isolation in a beautiful, fertile canyon-floor home.

About a week after arriving in Peach Springs and awakening each morning to the thunderous beauty of that place and its people, I knew I was home. Not the home that formed the context of my years growing up in New Jersey, but a spiritual home that I immediately felt.

Indian people are not a homogeneous group, despite what many bureaucrats in Washington would like to believe. Incorrectly called Indians, because Christopher Columbus went the wrong way in the Atlantic and thought he had stumbled on India, they are now known by the rational description Native Americans. Many Indians, however, feel that term, too, has an uncomfortable ring to it, and would rather be officially referred to by their modern tribal names—Navajo, Zuni, Cayuse, Cree, Nambe, for example—or by the traditional designation of Dine (Navajo) or Tohono O'odham (Papago). To each other, they call themselves "*in*-deuns," with a heavy accent on the initial sound.

Each tribe, band, pueblo, or nation is as dissimilar from any other as Germans are from Spanish, or British from Arabs. Each has its own unique culture, language, and environment, and strenuously objects to being lumped together with the others.

But for all the differences among tribes, there are many recurrent themes. Indian people are strongly respectful and protective of their traditions, many of which have been so diluted or destroyed that the integrity of the tribe itself is now at risk. They have an overriding concern for the strength of the extended family and for the protective, nurturing function of the tribe as a whole. Rarely are orphans found in a tribal group. No one goes hungry unless there is no food for anyone. As a group, these people have a deep, abiding respect for the earth—the mother, as they call it—from which all comes and all returns. And they honor a similar cosmology that depicts how the universe works, how the balance between spirit, mind, body, and the elements of the universe, such as wind, rocks, and animals, is intertwined in cycles of birth, death, and rebirth.

There are many reasons why Indian people suffer terribly from ill health. A majority of Indians are locked in abject poverty, and the unrelenting effects of impoverishment, lack of educational opportunities, and geographic isolation foster a cycle of illness, which is now commonplace. These are the obvious factors agreed upon by Indian people and by the federal agencies whose mandate it is to provide them with health and social services.

But the people themselves have other explanations that point out the difference between how Indians and non-Indians view the workings of the universe. Ask any tribal elder why their people suffer such distressing health statistics and they'll answer without hesitation that it's because the cultural harmony of the tribe has been lost. The sacred mountains where the medicine people went to gather healing plants are now in private hands, off-limits, with barbed wire preventing passage. The sacred sites of Indian ancestors are owned by the federal government and used for bombing ranges, or ski resorts, or privately operated mining concerns. The rivers where the salmon run are blockaded by hydroelectric dams producing electricity for the hairdryers of Los Angeles. The reasons for the disruption of the old ways, these elders will say, are many. But results are the same: because the harmony and balance so important to tribal integrity have been impaired, sickness has come to the people.

The sickness experienced by most tribes stretches across the spectrum of medical and traumatic disease. Diabetes is rampant among many groups, and malnutrition affects the young during those important growing years. Maternal and child death-rates, until quite recently, were many times above the national average.

It is in the world of trauma and psychosocial disease, however, that the greatest health risks now lie. The chances of a young Indian dying traumatically are three times the national average. Alcohol abuse is viewed by most Indians as their greatest problem, and its sequelae of violence, depression, suicide, and breakup of the all-important family structure has had perhaps the most devastating effects on the health of the people. Statistics in almost all categories except heart disease and cancer are markedly above national norms for non-Indians. Despite a self-sustaining legacy that abhors imbalances, both physical and spiritual, these have become a part of the modern Indian experience.

My personal memories are countless. I have delivered babies by lantern light in isolated log-and-mud homes, and have helped with a breech delivery of a calf in the middle of a spring snowstorm. I have seen isolated clinics run out of critically needed antibiotics at the height of flu season, and have watched dirt roads heading to health facilities become impassable during spring thaws. I have seen new clinics built and morbidity statistics turned around in selected areas. I have seen new generations come to birth and young friends succumb to violent deaths as a result of hopelessness and despair.

The Indian experience for which I was not prepared through my training was the world of traditional medicine. Some tribes, such as the Navajo and Tohono O'odham, have a strong and viable system of traditional healers who provide a substantial measure of health care alongside the "Western" medicine practiced by Indian Health Service workers. In many other tribes, however, much has been lost. For them, traditional medicine is not readily available, and is known only through stories told by elders late at night.

The basic tenet of all traditional medicine is that harmony between the body, the spirit, and the environment produces a state of wellness; if any of these elements are disrupted, a state of disharmony prevails and the person gets sick. This belief is more akin to traditional Oriental practices than to those taught in American or European medical schools. The role of the traditional healer is to "diagnose" (usually through divine means) what has caused an imbalance and then to restore the balance, using a wide variety of techniques including herbs, massage, day-long chanting-praying ceremonies called "sings," sweat baths, and the spiritual "transfer" of illness from patient to medicine person.

A number of tribes now utilize portions of both medical systems. The Tohono O'odham have well-documented traditional healing techniques that define illness as either "Indian" or "white man" sickness. If the causative agents are determined to be spiritual, the patient is sent to the medicine person first. If the sickness has been induced through Western influences, such as trauma or acute infection in a child, the patient is directed to the Indian Health Service hospital. This method of using the best of each health-care system has given the Tohono O'odham options unavailable to many smaller, more disenfranchised tribes.

I remember spending a day in the dusty central plaza of San Juan Pueblo in northern New Mexico. Traditions run strong in this pueblo, which has been continually inhabited for almost 400 years. It was the day of the Corn Dance, and the entire population was out in force, dressed in traditional garb, dancing in long lines of rhythmic movements as drummers kept up a hypnotic beat and elders sang traditional chants. Tourists lined the plaza, taking pictures of what seemed like a good show after having obtained the necessary pass and paid a fee to the tribal officers.

But the real purpose of the Corn Dance is not to entertain tourists. The dance has been traditionally performed to extend critical prayers and good energy to the spiritual forces in the universe that bring summer rains to this dry high-desert land so that the corn and other crops might grow and the people might survive another season. The dance has been performed for centuries, controlled rigidly in timing and content by the pueblo's spiritual leaders, who learned the ways passed on from generation to generation.

From this perspective, the dance was far from a show. The leather-clad feet of the dancers kicked up swirls of dust in the central plaza, where there had been no rain for weeks. The dancers had begun at dawn, and now late in the afternoon, after eight hours of almost continuous dancing and singing of timeless songs, high wispy clouds began to thicken and darken in the western sky. A cool wind came from the west, and most tourists began to retreat to their cars to return to Santa Fe.

The clouds turned black, and thunder clapped against the adobe mud walls of the pueblo. Then the rains came, nurturing the dry earth and bringing life to the dormant seeds the people had planted weeks before. Another season had come.

It was deemed a good dance. The proper energy had been expended, and balances once again restored. Such is the way of the people in this land.

Part Two

THE SEDUCTION
OF TRAUMA

(Fall 1979–Fall 1993)

*M*ore *by accident than by intent, I began practicing emergency medicine at a trauma center
in northern New Mexico. I eventually evolved into
becoming the emergency department medical director
and medical director for all EMS services in New
Mexico. Emergency medicine posed a strange dichoto-
my for me, for my style and respect for traditional
Indian medicine seemed in stark contrast to the loud,
animated, high-tech world of emergency medicine. But
the passion of emergency care, where immediacy had its
own seductive aura was real and gratifying, and kept
me emotionally captured for almost eighteen years.*

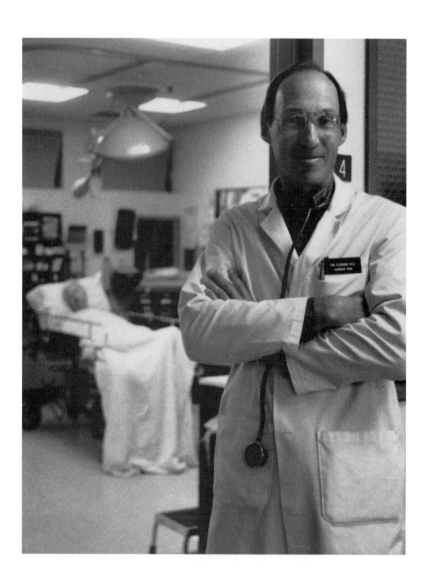

The Real ER

THE FIRST THING MOST PEOPLE NOTICE when entering an emergency room is the sounds. Babies cry incessantly in curtained cubicles. Moans of pain and fear—often from the elderly—come from unseen places. From the glass-enclosed, locked psychiatric holding room, muffled and guttural obscenities are hurled out to no one in particular. In other treatment areas, curses are heard from those getting injections or having fractures realigned. The phone rings unrelentingly, often going unanswered. The sounds, almost all harsh and disturbing, bounce off each other in a cacophony of uneasiness. As people enter this noisy milieu, they are struck at once by the fact that this is not a place of tranquillity.

The hospital emergency room is a place few ever choose to visit, but unfortunately becomes a necessary stop sometime during most people's lives. Often when people meet me in the "outside world" for the first time and hear what my work is, they say, "Boy, I hope never to see you in there." But see me they do, sooner or later. Having been in emergency medicine for almost seventeen years, I know that virtually everyone in Santa Fe County, either as a patient or accompanying one, has come through the doors of the local emergency room at least once.

The emergency room is a place dramatized in books, movies,

99

and a popular prime-time television series. The drama of life does indeed unfold in the ER, as those representations would have you believe. But it is not the sterile drama we experience in cinema, where scores die at the hands of a "terminator" though no one ever dies in a palpable way that disturbs us. In the ER, death is real and shocking in its ugliness, its finality. It isn't TV or the movies.

The emergency room at Santa Fe's only general hospital, St. Vincent, is a modern unit recently redesigned at the cost of a few million dollars. Its interior reminds some of the command deck of a starship, with high-tech monitors beeping and pulsating with colored patterns. A central nursing station serves as the hub to twenty-one rooms radiating out in all directions. The treatment areas run the range from large trauma and resuscitation rooms, where teams of staff often collide as they attempt to keep alive the critically ill and injured, to a number of single examination rooms with pale-curtain barriers to keep the outside world from intruding. Some are specialized for obstetrics and gynecology, others for pediatrics, and still others for orthopedic or laceration care.

Although the circular pattern of rooms coming off this central work station was designed to allow staff to simultaneously watch patients in multiple rooms, the arrangement has given rise to another phenomenon. From the entrance to each cubicle and examination room, anxious family members can stand and watch the scurrying of staff in the center, all the while asking themselves the same question: When will it be our turn to be seen? On a busy evening, the ER takes on the qualities of a gigantic fishbowl.

Because St. Vincent is the only general hospital in town, its ER is busy as hell. The facility is not only a formally designated Level II Trauma Center but also the standard referral hospital for much of northern New Mexico. So in addition to emergencies that pour through the doors from the streets and homes in Santa Fe County, on any given day St. Vincent's ER is also strained to capacity with patients from as far away as Taos, Clayton, and Chama.

The number of patient visits to the ER has increased steadily every year for the last decade. Between the emergency room itself and its adjacent urgent care center (designed to treat simple medical problems not needing the full resources of the ER), St. Vincent sees more than 50,000 patients a year. That's second in the state only to the University Hospital in Albuquerque for number of ER visits.

The name "emergency room" is a misnomer, for it is neither just one room nor the site of only emergency care. To those who work there, it is more reasonably referred to as the emergency department, for its complexity supports that broader description. But its well-known initials— ER—are as deeply ingrained in the populace as other common shortcuts such as IRS or NBA. So, ER it remains.

And true to its name, it does experience the full spectrum of emergencies: the critical auto crashes, the stabbings and shootings, the heart attacks, and the children in sudden respiratory distress. But unfortunately, its major load is cases that could more easily be seen in other settings: people with chronic abdominal pain or headaches, the hundreds who come through the doors each day with simple upper respiratory infections or the flu, and even those with minor ailments who cannot get in to see their own doctor, or just as commonly, have no physician or health insurance, and use the ER as their primary source of health care when illness hits between the eyes.

The overcrowded ERs of many urban settings, bursting with masses of real and unreal emergencies, have been highlighted by some as the symbolic focal point for "everything wrong with the US health-care system." Too many people without resources or health coverage crowd into the ER at the last minute when their medical problems— which could have been mitigated through preventive care—have worsened to the point of true emergencies.

Walk into any big-city ER and you face a quagmire of people needing care, and not enough rooms or staff to stem the tide. Those sick enough to require hospital admission will often be kept in the ER for hours to days until inpatient beds, filled to capacity, gradually open up. Some patients never get to leave the ER for that needed admission, but instead die quietly in the cubicles and back hallways while waiting for a bed to become available.

At St. Vincent, as well as most hospitals in New Mexico, those urban problems of overcrowding and waiting times of up to ten hours are a rarity. But depending on when one arrives at the doors, the wait can still be intolerable and confusing. Everyone who "presents" feels he or she has an emergency. It's simply that some emergencies take preference over others. When the beds in the ER are filled with those still being treated or waiting for admission, and the ambulances continue to arrive like commercial jets in a holding pattern at O'Hare, the waiting room becomes a place where patience wears thin. Those automatic double doors leading into the inner sanctum, offering a promise of relief and attention, rarely open often enough to those still waiting.

Chris has been at it for longer than he cares to remember. (In the ER only first names appear on identification tags. That's so that some distraught person cannot try to find an ER worker at home later on.) One of the staff of emergency medicine physicians working at the hospital, Chris has seen it all and felt the chaos of the ER with its unrelenting intensity. He was trained in family practice, but came to emergency medicine almost fourteen years ago. He, like all ER physicians at St. Vincent, is board certified in the relatively new specialty of emergency medicine—something that is not true of a lot of hospitals, as a recent nationwide report made clear.

It is a rare breed that can do this work of moving within moments from critical cardiac care to psychiatrist, to pediatrician, to facial surgeon, all the while trying to juggle the surge of patients coming through the doors. But despite the excitement of the work, there remain lingering frustrations. "What gets to me sometimes," Chris says quietly, "is all the stuff that comes in with the patient and what they present you with. The complaint—be it headache or stomach pain—is just the tip of the iceberg. It's always just a manifestation of other things: the unhappiness in their lives, the hassles at work, and all the rest. In the ER, we just don't have time to get to the bottom of what's really happening. We don't have time to really deal with things."

The camaraderie he feels working with others in the ER is of special significance. "In this place," he says, "we're all in it together. It doesn't matter what your title is or what degree you have, everyone—the EKG techs, the phlebotomists, the nurses—is in this together."

After all his years in this arena, Chris has come to realize something important about the human condition. "Here we often see people at the lowest point in their lives, whether it was caused by them or others. Here they are naked," he says. "And even though they've sunk to the depths, we've seen it all and accept them without judgment. I think that really helps in what we do."

Chris does realize that his work is a young person's profession. Now in his mid-forties, when not working in the ER or coming off a night shift, he actively pursues vigorous endeavors like biking, volleyball, skiing, and exercising at the gym. He admits he can see spending only another five to ten years in the high-pressure world of emergency medicine. "I think I can do this until I'm fifty," he says. "Maybe even fifty-five. But it's something you can't do when you're sixty."

Then there is Patti. She, too, has been working in the ER for most of her adult life. A nurse for twenty-three years and at St. Vincent's ER for the past seventeen, she has earned the rank of veteran, and with it the respect and affection of everyone in the facility. Her small frame and soft voice give comfort to patients when they need that caring touch. But any patient who becomes aggressive or abusive gets her loud Irish-Massachusetts brogue right in their face. She is not to be trifled with.

Patti has attempted the difficult change that crosses the minds of many who work in the ER: to escape its stressful environment and move on to something more peaceful, more measured. She has tried to escape not once, but twice, only to return to the ER each time. She tried a stint as a nurse in the coronary care unit. A number of years later, she took a job with the AIDS Wellness Center. As appealing as each new experience was, she missed the intensity of the ER too much.

"I left both times because of frustration," she says. "You know, that place is both physically and emotionally hard on you. It takes its toll. I just kept thinking there was something more interesting I could do."

The reason she returned? "I found I really missed the reality of the ER—I mean, it's so real, what we do. The people we help cross all social and economic barriers. Everyone is equal, and the problems they have are real. Despite all the machines we use, our work comes down to the people and their real problems."

The feeling of family among the staff also helped draw her back. "I found I missed the people there too much. What an incredible group they are. That's what makes it so special," she says softly. "They all accept each other and the patients for simply who they are."

For everyone who has worked emergency rooms for years, there remain memories of those types of cases that raise the flow of adrenalin, no matter how callous and hardened we think we might be. For some, it's the critically ill babies, so helpless in their tired cries, so unable to communicate how they feel. For others, it's the spouses and children abused by family members. For still others, it's the often unrepentant ones who have just caused fatal injuries through the negligence of drinking and driving.

For me and many others, it is the trauma cases that linger the most—the auto crashes, stabbings, shootings, beatings. Trauma has its own inherent karma that speaks of violence and blood and frightening randomness.

There are usually one or two cases that remain fixed in the memories of the emergency room staff no matter how much time has passed since they enveloped us in their moment. These memories are life dreams that come back as readily as the nightmares of war.

My recurrent memories are three:

• The 1980 New Mexico prison riot, in which more than thirty inmates were brutally murdered and hundreds of others, both guards and inmates, critically injured. I was staffing the ER for almost thirty hours of that weekend siege, which quickly took on surreal overtones. What lingers is not so much individual cases, but the lasting feeling that the event symbolized both man's inhumanity to man as well as the nature of our society that drives people to commit such acts of utter hopelessness.

• The young man, an acquaintance and member of my softball team, who was brought to the ER one night having attempted suicide by pressing a rifle under his chin. He had only partially succeeded, removing most of his face in the process. His widely spaced eyes, still receiving visual input as we frantically worked on him, looked at me with a bizarre wonder and confusion that will always haunt me.

• The four-year-old boy who, having just lost his mother in an auto crash, was spied by me standing utterly alone in a back hallway of the ER, unable to cry, processing thoughts I couldn't even begin to imagine.

The immediacy of those traumatic moments rarely affects one while at work. ER staffers, through training and experience, have learned the important lesson of burying the emotional content of those draining events while on duty, aware that the patients who continue to need care deserve someone who is collected and functional.

But the thoughts do return—usually when one gets off work and begins to unwind at home or with friends at a watering hole. The thoughts and the need to talk about them do not get dealt with easily. They rarely get ventilated sufficiently with spouses, friends, and workers. The ER staff, as individuals, all deal with the stress of the work in their own ways—some healthy, some less so. For many, the place understandably takes its toll in spirit, and they move on to different things. Others find a way to cope with seeing the nakedness so acutely, and remain in the passionate arena for many years—hating those troublesome moments, yet delighting in the intensity of it all.

But life in the ER is not only sadness and troublesome memories. This is part of the contradiction of that environment, and the reason people like Chris and Patti and all the others continue to work there despite the unbelievable stress it can produce. For every child with a critical head injury, there is a new baby born in the OB room. For every draining case, there are more who get better, are unburdened of their suffering moment, and reward you with a smile of appreciation. There are so many who are helped, so much pain and fear relieved, so many lives saved. Those moments are what keep the staff rejuvenated in the work they do.

The ER. It's a place of drama, chaos, and contradiction—and now it's on network television in prime time. Let's hope the Hollywood version of that world does justice to the women and men who choose to be there for real, ready to help when the nasty sirens begin screaming down our streets.

The Night Shift

 THE ROUND CLOCK ON THE WALL on at the nurses' station reads 2:05 A.M. Can it really be this far into the morning? I ask myself.

I stop writing on the medical chart in front of me and stare again at the white dial—the instrument that seems to mark these long twelve-hour shifts in the emergency room. Rarely do I glance at it early in the shift, but as the hours press on and my sense of finishing off seems less tangible, all that changes. My sense of time during a night shift is stepped off initially in hours, then in fifteen-minute intervals, and finally, in agonizing minutes that seem to drag on eternally between seven and nine in the morning.

Thus far, this Friday night–Saturday morning shift has been busy, though not unmanageable. The bars are now beginning to close. Last call for drinks has long passed. Most wild parties have long since fizzled out, and the bulk of teenagers are at home, having survived the journey through city streets to the warmth and safety of their beds. Men and women struggling with the deep pain of madness or depression either have already fallen asleep or are locked in with loved ones who are used to their frantic nighttime calls for help. No major auto crashes have sent screaming, traumatized patients pouring in through the emergency room doors. No fights, no stabbings, no shootings. What a strangely quiet Friday night, I think, taking a moment to reflect on all that has happened.

I had arrived, as usual, by 9:00 P.M. While others were wending their way home and settling into bed, I was driving through the nighttime chill to the hospital on the south side of town. The streets were filled with traffic—after all, it was date night, the end of the workweek, and payday. While passing the drivers as they moved slowly out from the center of town, I found myself going through my preshift ritual wondering how many of them would find their way, by choice or fate, to our emergency room as the night wore on.

The emergency center was filled to capacity when I arrived. Every stretcher and cubicle was occupied with someone needing care. Six untouched charts still hung on the board by the clock. Doctors and nurses were moving rapidly around the central station, their voices raised in pressured speech, their clipboards thrown hastily on the desk. Family members of patients stood in entrances to the exam rooms, staring relentlessly at the nurses' station and wondering when the doctor would be in, when the lab tests would be back.

Typically, it does not seem frantic when I arrive at work. I feel excited entering the fray relatively rested and bright-eyed, as though it's the opening tip-off and the next hours might open wide with hundreds of provocative events. The day at home had been leisurely enough; I'd caught up on chores around the house, watched a new video release, and grabbed a few hours of deep sleep in the late afternoon. So naturally, coming through the large double-glass doors at the ambulance entrance and seeing that chaos of humanity got my blood pumping and my hormones coursing, as is often true.

As it turned out, many difficult and complex "cases" were still waiting to be seen. My day-shift colleagues had been at it for over twelve hours and wanted desperately to finish off charts and head out the doors to other worlds. Some would go home to their families whereas others, off to the local pubs, would meet with fellow hospital staff to quickly imbibe and unwind.

I began to rapidly process these patients who were waiting. An elderly woman who lived up in the mountains to the north was lying on a gurney stretcher, surrounded by half a dozen concerned family members who, having made their monthly visit to her that day, had found her huddled in bed—pale and breathless, for she had not eaten in two days. They wanted quick answers, an instant understanding of why "Grandmother" was ill. They wanted her in the hospital "just for a rest," not realizing that the doors to this expensive motel do not swing open freely. Aware of the shortage of beds and nursing staff, of the concern that the hospital would not be reimbursed by Medicare for a noncritical admission, and of the difficulty in finding an internist or family practitioner willing to take on a new patient, I knew that getting her admitted would be an alley fight. I did not immediately share this troublesome reality with the family, since it would not have helped them overcome their frustration. Instead, I ordered a battery of laboratory tests, X rays, and ECGs, hoping that enough imbalances found in the frail grandmother's metabolic milieu would make her admission an easy sell to the internist on call.

The orthopedic room was packed with six patients. Most had fallen or twisted a joint during the day and thought little of it until bedtime when the deep, throbbing pain of engorged joint capsules and ligaments had shaken them from sleep. X rays were ordered, splints applied, crutches measured, and narcotic medicines dispensed. Before long, the room was cleared and my sense of accomplishment moved forward.

Two youngsters with facial lacerations were awaiting in adjoining cubicles. Their stories were familiar: in the last frantic moments before the little ones had rejected the inevitability of bedtime, with its darkened rooms and potential for bad dreams, they'd been bouncing on sofas and chasing around coffee tables when a slip occurred, a cheek caught the edge of a table, and the unblemished flesh was rent amid a scream of pain and blood. To the parents, there is the fear of enduring scars that will forever assign their precious one to a life of rejection. To the kids, the smell of antiseptics and moans from unseen patients in adjacent treatment areas suggest that this is a frightening place, a place to be cautious and fearful.

Between reassuring the parents, calming their kids, and freeing up enough staff to hold the little bodies still, I was able to approach their moving targets on cheeks and chins to repair the lacerations. Each took over thirty minutes, however, and by the time the sterile surgical gloves were removed and the wounds bandaged, six new patients had arrived. A sense of not getting ahead began to flow into me like venom from a familiar demon destined to be my companion for the next seven hours. Always, there is another patient to be seen . . . no end in sight.

A young woman lies in the gynecology room, tearful and afraid, for she has begun bleeding heavily partway into her third month of pregnancy. Her teenage boyfriend is holding her hand, looking lost and confused about his role in all this. A quick exam gives the impression she is experiencing a threatened miscarriage yet the pregnancy is still viable. Much time is spent reassuring, advising, conveying details about this process, and how at such an early stage, all of modern medicine cannot change what will happen naturally. She finally leaves for home, committed to lying in bed for days to help protect her fetus.

Now more pediatric cases begin lining up. A brother-sister pair come in, having awakened with the frightening bark and struggle for breath typical of the croup. But the speeding car ride through the cool and moist night air has already released the spasm from their vocal cords, and at this point the two youngsters are breathing easily, laughing at all the attention coming their way. After treating several children with fevers, coughs, and vomiting in the next room, I check on the elderly grandmother's lab tests—which confirm early renal failure, a problem serious enough to arrange for her admission, so I update her chart and look at the round clock on the wall . . . 4:30 A.M. The time has sped by. No new charts are hanging on the wall. Convinced the rush has now ended for the night, I am drawn even further back in time, wondering what brought me to this busy emergency department in the first place.

When the early 1970s, years of medical school and internship, left me undecided on any specialty, I joined the US Public Health Service and began an exciting, often draining seven years of living and working with various Indian tribes in Arizona, New Mexico, and Oregon. Right away, I took on a full spectrum of roles from clinician to social worker to administrator to occasional veterinarian. I then moved fully into administrative work operating Indian health systems in isolated settings, and eventually assisting the larger, more politically sophisticated Navajo and O'odham Nations in their attempts to improve health care for their people.

By the late 1970s, I was operating a small health consultant firm out of New Mexico and traveling extensively to meet with tribes throughout the Southwest. To make financial ends meet, however, and to satisfy my growing need to again wear "the white coat" and touch patients, I decided to work an occasional night shift at the local hospital's emergency room.

As time passed, this clinical involvement grew from two or three times a month to a full-time immersion in emergency medicine. The Indian consultant work became much less active. I joined a professional corporation that operated three emergency departments in northern New Mexico, and became a medical director for EMS programs involved in fire department and other emergency care services. After a long series of written and oral examinations, I then became board certified in emergency medicine. It was a career I never thought I would have, and it was all-consuming.

Throughout those years, I honed my emergency care skills to a sharp edge. Before long, I was equally at home treating critical medical and trauma cases, performing delicate plastic surgery, diagnosing pediatric infections, and intervening in psychiatric crises. I even developed pride in this medical career that was more incidental than planned.

There were voids, however, in the crisis-oriented work. I missed the extended interactions with patients and their families that had allowed me not only to provide immediate care but to assist in sorting through the complex social factors that play such an integral part in a person's illness. I missed the home visits, the doctoring of horses and cattle, and the connectedness that arises for a family physician practicing in a small, isolated community. I especially yearned for my work with Indian people, whose dignity, quiet ways, and sense of humor had made every interaction something special.

As for the ER, it was all fire and blood and urgency—plugging up dikes after physical or emotional collapse, offering interim resuscitation en route to the OR, or applying temporary bandages until more definitive care could be taken in the inpatient environment. Little human connectedness was possible—or even acceptable—for one had to be cool, competent, and ready to do major battle against threats to life and limb. This was high-tech medicine at its most intense. Moreover, patients were referred to by their pathology rather than their name. The staff would speak of "That open fracture in room twenty," "The incomplete miscarriage in number seven," and "The acute myocardial infarct in bed three." The focus was on problems, not complex people with special circumstances, unique perspectives, and hidden fears.

My reveries have been interrupted by cyclic rushes of four to five patients at once. At the moment a number of young adults with complex medical problems requiring extensive workups keep me from escaping to the small and odorous on-call room down the hall—a room that rarely sees use of its old hospital bed for catnaps during these shifts. The number of cups of bitter coffee I've downed from the stained pot in the nurses' lounge is beginning to approach double digits. I can feel my stomach and esophagus recoiling from the insult of caffeine and stale doughnuts.

At about 6:00 A.M., as I begin fantasizing about an escape out the back door to head home for sleep, a tearful young woman is brought in by friends. She was at a party last evening, and following one precipitous event after another, she accepted a ride home from a stranger who mistakenly thought her "no, no" meant "yes, yes" and forcibly raped her. She then sat at home for hours, shaking and crying uncontrollably until she found the strength to call friends. Sexual assault cases are invariably draining on me, requiring a difficult interplay between dealing with the Rape Crisis team, reporting to the police, obtaining necessary physical evidence, and treating the injuries, all the while trying to provide as much comfort to the victim as possible. As if this were not challenging enough, the support needs to be delicately balanced with the reality that I am a strange man who must examine her for injuries and obtain specimens from her most intimate places right after she has been horribly violated by another male stranger.

The last hour of the shift moves on with a painful slowness. As several new patients come through the doors, I surrender to the time-honored tradition of getting an initial history, doing a workup, ordering lab tests, and turning the case over to my replacement, who will soon be bouncing brightly through the doors.

Once back in the on-call room, I finish up the last of the charts. Often at this point in the progression of sleep deprivation, patients blur into one another. Was it the lady in room 3 or the motor crash victim who had the palpable lump on the right side? Which one had the abnormal blood pressure? My numb mind struggles to remember hundreds of complex variables stored there over the past twelve hours— hoping that I assign the right numbers to the appropriate patient.

At the end of these night shifts, when I'm finally free of patient responsibilities, I inevitably find myself "hanging around" the emergency room for a while. I sit by the nurses' station downing another cup of coffee, watching the brisk morning pace of incoming patients, and listening to the high-pressured dialogues back and forth between doctors, nurses, and techs. Despite all the hours spent trying to escape out the back door to return home for needed rest, I cling to this chaotic environment—as if in leaving it, I will leave behind a critical piece of myself that exults in caregiving in the midst of crisis.

Willie Angel

 WE LOST WILLIE ANGEL THE OTHER DAY.

Willie Angel—such a strange name for a bear of a man who looked anything but angelic. His big, round face, his bushy mustache, and the twinkling dark eyes behind his thick glasses spoke more of mischief than piety. He liked his off-colored jokes, his partying with friends and family, and when Willie slid up to the bar at his local FOB lodge, the bartender checked his supply of beer in the walk-in to make sure enough cases were on hand.

Willie Angel was a veteran police officer. Throughout his forty-two years, he burned bright and touched everyone he came in contact with, but the radiance took its toll. Willie died of a heart attack in the early morning hours. Despite all efforts of his paramedic pals in the fire department and staff at the emergency department, his heart couldn't be jump-started this time.

At his funeral, the city poured forth with its collective tears of loss. Not an empty pew could be found in the church, and there were standing-room-only crowds all the way out to the street. Not a dry eye in the house. Not one person who wasn't touch by this amazing man's warmth and love.

Willie had worked his way up the ranks in the police department after his time in the military. For years as a uniformed officer, and later as a detective with the juvenile division, he was the epitome of a cop who cared. Despite his rank, he missed "the streets and the people," so he returned to uniform a few years back and headed the traffic division. You could always see Willie on the streets around town—consoling auto-crash victims, talking to teenagers who should have been in school, and yes, helping little old ladies cross the street.

When he wasn't on duty, Willie was supporting a worthwhile cause of one sort or another. Each time a group sprang up to help kids in trouble, Willie was there to serve on the board and give whatever was necessary to keep the program alive. In recent years he spent most evenings at the Battered Women's Shelter, bringing a measure of joy to the kids and women in their time of greatest need. In short, he gave far more to improving human happiness than he took for himself.

Willie spent a great deal of time in our emergency department. No sooner would an ambulance pull in than he would be on the scene with a smile, a joke, or a story to lighten the atmosphere and prevent depression from setting in. His infectious style would force us to keep a positive perspective and move on to help the next person. Because of him, we learned not to remain mired in the tragedies that already took so much out of us.

Willie loved those who gave to others, especially Emergency Medical Technicians (EMTs) and nurses who, he said, made the world a better place than he ever could. Because of his admiration for EMTs, he made special efforts to learn all he could about emergency care, eventually becoming a certified first responder and cardiopulmonary resuscitation (CPR) instructor. Constantly, he challenged his fellow police officers to stay current on their first aid and CPR skills.

After his passing, nearly everyone in town had a Willie Angel story to tell. My personal story for Willie goes like this:

One Saturday evening about a year ago, Willie was volunteering his time at the senior citizens' dance downtown. The large ballroom was filled with elders happy to see old friends, share stories, and kick up their heels to salsa rhythms. Willie was there to make sure everyone had a good time and to dance with those little ladies who had no partners. Suddenly, a sixty-eight-year-old woman collapsed to the floor, and Willie was one of the first to reach her. No breath passed through her lips, no pulse could be found. Willie told someone to call 911 and then began administering CPR. The paramedic unit arrived in about six minutes to find the woman in ventricular fibrillation. Although it took a number of jolts to reverse the rhythm, she responded and was transported quickly to the hospital. Two weeks later she walked out of the hospital eager to attend the next senior citizens' dance.

I saw Willie the following day. He was beside himself with joy, because despite the countless people he had helped over the years as a police officer and community volunteer, never had he felt so fulfilled. Willie believed this was his most special moment.

It wasn't until a few months later, in the midst of a cold winter night when Willie and I found ourselves alone at the hospital, that I unexpectedly got an insight into why he had felt so transformed by resuscitating that woman. We were engaged in general gossip when he almost hypnotically lapsed into a deep-seated memory. His voice became soft and monotonal. Although details of his story were indistinct and difficult to follow, he spoke about an old problem in his extended family: a relative, saddled by his own demons, had suggested that Willie was into police work for the delusion of power, that any mission to help others was a selfish facade. There seemed to be other painful memories surfacing as well, but Willie's rendering of them were indistinct and confusing. He was only able to speak of his personal pain while lost in thought, then frightened by the intensity of the feelings returning to him, he would abruptly change the subject. He never mentioned these matters to me again.

Still, I have the overwhelming sense that Willie had begun to venture into those locked closets of personal experience that we all possess. Their contents, once discovered, are rarely if ever shared with family, spouse, or others who are emotionally important to us. The stuff of deep secret, they are tapped only by chance when something incredible enters our lives—something like breathing renewed life into a human being who is slipping away.

When Willie Angel died suddenly at age forty-two, my silent prayer to him included thanks—for reminding me that we all have those pockets of personal experience, that they are not the province of anyone else. After all, these strands of mystery help define our uniqueness.

The Escape
Place

FOR ALMOST SEVENTEEN YEARS NOW I've been practicing
emergency medicine at St. Vincent Hospital in the northern
mountains of New Mexico. There is an old adage that
such work is a young person's profession. After a few night shifts, I am
convinced this saying holds great truth.

The emergency room is often tumultuous, frequently theatrical,
and almost always stressful. There we not only face sudden life-and-
death events—the heart attacks and gunshots—but also serve as a
refuge for people who don't have a doctor of their own, can't get an
appointment, or have a real or imagined emergency after-hours.

Typically, our circular emergency room is filled to capacity with
patients of every age and medical problem. Permeating the air are cries
of frightened babies, moans of adults with abdominal pain, and that
ever-present question issuing forth from each cubicle: "When am I
going to be seen?" Even on the rare occasions when the ER is not busy,
the anticipation of an emergency coming through the door can be
enormously stressful. Staff are chronically tired, biorhythms are out of
whack, and insanity reigns supreme.

Consequently, when I can get away, I escape to a place of healing. At such times I seek a setting that is tranquil instead of chaotic,

blessedly quiet instead of cacophonous, and peaceful rather than confrontational.

Most often I head for a place on Santa Clara Pueblo land, near their ancestral ruins at Puyé Cliffs. The drive itself is relaxing. After crossing the muddy Rio Grande at Otowi Bridge, I watch the multicolored mesas and canyons of the Jémez Mountains spread out before me. Always, the play of shadows and colors is different.

Near Puyé Cliff ruins, I break off onto a forest road heading south. Depending on the season and road conditions (snow and mud often make too much adventure impossible), I will find a spot back among the pines, with views of the ochre-colored, pockmarked Puyé Cliffs peeking through the trees. It is a gentle place where light winds usually whisper through the ponderosa, juniper, and piñon. Eagles and hawks often glide silently overhead, looking for quarry in the canyons below.

When the roads are passable, I'll travel farther into the Jémez toward Guaje Canyon. Here the forest roads tend to be treacherous, with deep ruts from melting snows and sharp rocks jutting up, ready to render any tire suddenly useless. The winding and intersecting trails eventually merge with the forest. I then go by foot another mile or so up to an isolated mesa top once shown to me by a close friend who had studied petroglyphs, or ancient rock art, in the area.

On that thin finger of a mesa is an unexcavated Anasazi ruin. The old pueblo walls have since crumbled into chest-high mounds of earth completely covered with grasses and small piñons. Pot shards of various sizes, many bearing painted patterns, litter the dry earth. The quietness at this place has an almost musical quality. It feels timeless and infused with a gentle spirit.

At the end of the finger of land, before the earth falls off a few hundred feet to the canyon below, one can sit facing east and see the entire expanse of the Sangre de Cristo Mountains—from beyond Albuquerque's Manzano peaks to the south all the way to Wheeler Peak and the Colorado border to the north. You have to stare hard to see any signs of civilization in the valley below.

I often sit on this lip of land and lose myself in harmony until time ceases to matter. At that point the emergency room, far from being a distant memory, no longer exists. Only the sky, the earth, and the thunderous quiet are real.

The Pen Riot

ON FEBRUARY 2, 1980, the Penitentiary of New Mexico, near Santa Fe, erupted in two days of horrible rioting, burning, and murder as overcrowded inmates lashed out at the hopelessness they felt in confinement. When the facility was peacefully retaken thirty-six hours later, the horror of what had occurred behind those walls began to unfold. The author was on duty as the physician in charge of the local hospital's emergency department during those two days of massacre. This remembrance was written soon after the last patient was treated and life in the hospital had begun to return to normal.

A sea of people clustered around the central station. Nurses in white, respiratory therapists in green surgical gowns, city police, National Guardsmen, security forces with walkie-talkies all clustered around the small nurses' station in the emergency department straining to hear static-filled transmissions over the emergency radio. Off to the side, some people talked quietly of other things. But for most, their attention was riveted on the radio chatter.

It was the second day of the infamous inmate takeover at the Penitentiary of New Mexico, that explosive event that had captured the lives and concerns of people throughout New Mexico and the country. For two days, inmates at the horribly overcrowded maximum-security facility south of Santa Fe had gone on an unexplainable rampage of destruction, death, and mayhem. After it was over, thirty-three inmates were found dead, many having been brutally tortured by other inmates. Hundreds of prisoners and guards, as well, were injured or critically affected by drug overdoses. The facility was virtually destroyed and required expensive rebuilding. More importantly, the riot shook the consciousness of this quiet rural state where the pace of life is slow and the concerns of people more aligned with agrarian matters than with urban violence.

From the smoke-filled air around the prison, critically injured guards and inmates were being transported to the closest medical facility—the one community hospital in Santa Fe. The emergency entrance on the building's northwest side became a dramatic stage where anxious relatives collected to catch a glimpse of loved ones being rushed inside.

Since the early-dawn hours on Saturday, the causalities had been coming in—slowly at first, just three inmates and one guard. Then as the day wore on and more injured were brought from interior cell blocks to the prison's perimeter, wave after wave of emergency transports were rushed to the hospital.

The most critical cases came by National Guard helicopter, a massive Army-green Huey that shattered the air with the thud-thud-thud of its whirling blades. Others were rushed over by ambulance or hastily thrown in the back of police cars. Although the National Guard medical staff at the prison tried to exercise some control over transporting the injured, from the perspective of those at the hospital, patients seemed to simply come in waves—one after another, all day Saturday, then through the nighttime hours, and again all day Sunday. Almost an unrelenting onslaught, like a MASH unit in Vietnam.

For the emergency department personnel and support staff from the hospital clustered around the radio that afternoon, the crisis at the penitentiary was taking an inevitable toll on their energies. Nothing like it had ever happened to them before.

There was something bizarre, something surrealistic about the sound of helicopters cutting through the air above, the sight of men with loaded M-16 rifles walking past litters of patients lined up like pieces of beef in the hallways, and the stench of foul smoke on clothes and in the air. But most draining of all to those there that day was the incessant uncertainty of the situation.

Weekends at that hospital were typically busy, with a steady stream of survivors of auto crashes, fights, and the occasional stabbing around town. Yet aside from streaks of bad nights, there remained a steady-state atmosphere to the emergencies in that place. People came in, were treated, and then the quiet moments would return.

But that Sunday was different. There was seemingly no end to the waves of injured appearing at the prison's perimeter. The siege was in its second day, with no sign of successful negotiations. Smoke continued to pour from the prison into the crisp winter air of high-altitude Santa Fe.

Although the emergency department had seen and treated almost 100 patients from the crisis, ten times that number were still entrapped in that hysteria-laden and explosive situation—bleeding and maimed men who could, at any moment, suddenly appear at the emergency department entrance if the crisis ever escalated into a bloody assault on the smoldering penitentiary.

It was that uncertainty and sense of endless casualties that began to grip the staff on Sunday afternoon. For thirty hours everyone had been working frantically yet efficiently—moving patients from helicopters to the emergency ward, and then on to admission throughout the hospital. But in the early afternoon, as people began crowding around the radio for more information from the prison, the rarely spoken rumors began spreading. "The National Guard is going to storm the place . . . Negotiations have broken down . . . Expect heavy casualties at any time . . ."

It was then that the faces of those tired medical staff took on a blankness of despair not seen before. Talk became less frequent and the regular joking back and forth stopped, as if everyone were asking a silent question: "If what we have seen the last two days is only the tip of the iceberg, what can we do when it really blows up?"

The previous day had been easier. There was a seductive newness to the experience of being in a disaster situation in which all resources of the community were mobilized to deal with sudden crisis. Extra staff had poured into the hospital—some who had been called in from home, and many more who simply stopped by, volunteering to help out as best they could. On that first day, no one was sure of the injuries expected or how long the crisis would last. There was a high level of energy and almost intoxicating, heady excitement in the air.

The first major rush of injured from the prison did not immediately quell that high. Primarily victims of smoke inhalation from fires raging since early morning hours, the initial patients were not seriously ill, and with oxygen therapy and quick evaluation, almost all were well enough to be returned to the prison holding area, now entrenched with security forces.

It was not until these first patients reached the safety of the hospital and began hesitantly talking that the true scope of the catastrophe began to unfold. There were stories of inmates who refused to join the riot being mercilessly beaten and tortured by other prisoners. Vendettas against opposing gang members were taking place constantly. Others told tales of men jumping through glass windows and down elevator shafts to escape attacks by marauding groups of rioters. They were tales of a world gone mad, a nightmare of darkness, smoke, screams, and utter despair that there no longer seemed a human soul left in some rioters. The faces of those patients were locked in masks of fear, their voices quivering as they tried to speak.

"I've just been prayin' to the Lord since last night," one burly black inmate said. "Just prayin' and prayin' that I wouldn't be killed."

Another said, "I haven't prayed in thirty years, but since last night, I've been praying for them to spare me." He then began to cry uncontrollably.

Still another inmate, a middle-aged man from the southern part of the state who had been at the prison barely three days, undergoing an evaluation period for a petty offense, was lying on a stretcher rubbing his swollen and discolored lower leg. It had been injured when he jumped through a plate-glass window trying to escape the mobs of club-wielding inmates. "I never thought people could act that way . . . I don't understand how they could," he murmured, before breaking into sobs.

Over the next hours, the types of casualties brought to the hospital changed dramatically, confirming the horrors told by other prisoners. Men who had been brutally beaten began to appear, many with stab wounds of the face, neck, and chest. An inmate with a partially severed arm from an attack with a meat cleaver was wheeled through the door. All were serious but treatable, and were stabilized as well as possible before being quickly moved on to operating rooms or intensive care units.

Stories began to filter over to the hospital about inmates who wouldn't need to be transported. As if compelled to demonstrate the horror of life behind the walls, some rioters had begun to ritualistically bring to the perimeter area bodies of those already dead. Decapitations, dismembered bodies, those killed by torture. The hospital staff never saw these patients, but stories of them were whispered back and forth, intensifying the agony.

Soon there appeared men who had taken massive drug overdoses. The rioters had broken into the prison infirmary, and in a frenzy had taken every possible combination of pills, liquids, and injections. "We're getting a rush of overdoses out here now," yelled the National Guard medic over the radio from the prison grounds. "We've got some serious situations out here." And in they came, sometimes three at a time from the helicopter.

Most were seriously unconscious, with barely enough spontaneous breathing to sustain themselves. Each was rushed into the emergency department, quickly stabilized, and moved to a hospital floor for more specialized treatment. New litters were opened up for the next wave of overdoses. A nurse went from stretcher to stretcher with a felt-tip marker placing identification numbers on their chests: John Doe 13 . . . John Doe 14.

Finally, late Sunday afternoon, after more than thirty-two hours of constant activity, word began to spread through the emergency department that the police had taken control of the prison compound. No shots had been exchanged. The feared onslaught of wounded inmates and guardsmen would not be materializing. More injuries would be coming in, but not with the severity or in the numbers that had been dreaded.

By six that evening, the crisis seemed over. Most staffers who had packed the department all those hours had now disappeared, leaving the area frighteningly deserted and tranquil. The usual trickle of Sunday evening emergency patients then began to appear. As quickly as the crisis had developed, it dissolved, as if little had happened. One last helicopter transport of four patients was to come in that evening, but the problems were quickly resolved and pace soon returned to normal.

Even so, an overwhelming sense of sadness lingered after the last evacuation helicopter left. Merged with the sadness was helplessness in understanding what it had all been about. Only as the next days unfolded would the true story of horror and inhumanity at the penitentiary become known. In the emergency department those two days, only a glimmer of that thunderous human agony had been felt, yet the gloom it left behind remained.

The events of those thirty-six hours in that hospital's emergency department went far beyond the usual trauma to the human soul. It had all been too massive, too unbelievable to comprehend. It had broken all the rules.

This story was first printed in The Santa Fe Reporter *and later received the 1980 Guy Rader Award, sponsored annually by the New Mexico Medical Society to recognize "excellent reporting in the field of health." In the eighteen years that had passed since the initiation of the Rader Award, the author was the first winner who was also a doctor.*

Wonder in the ER

I HESITATE BEFORE THE DOOR leading to that small room. Although the people inside have never seen me before, I'm about to give them the worst news they have ever heard. I'm about to change their lives forever, and they don't know me from the man who stacks their groceries every Friday.

I take a deep breath, reminding myself I've done this before—too many times to count. As soon as I enter the room, their eyes lock on me. I'm wearing my white coat and other garb of the profession, so they know I'm official, I think to myself. During a quick round of introductions, I make a mental note of the family connections: the wife here, a few grown children in the corner, an elderly brother by the far wall.

The telling comes quickly and directly: "I'm terribly sorry, but it appears he suffered a major and massive event. The paramedics did all they could. We tried everything we know how in the emergency room, but we just couldn't start his heart again. I'm sorry, but he's gone."

The familiar announcement flows easily from my lips. I inject it with enough concern to avoid conveying too much coldness. But I didn't know the man, and I don't know these people. I can't cry with them, for I had no connection. I am simply the messenger.

Then I pay close attention—and I wonder—as the response unfolds from this gathering of stunned people. Sure, we watch movies and daytime soaps; we read romantic novels; hence we think we have some sense of how unfair fate can be. But how do we react when the unspeakable, the unacceptable suddenly strikes us between the eyes? The fabric of this family's life has just been ripped apart, sent swirling into an oblique well of loss and confusion.

I wonder at their responses. For some, there are tears; for others, screams of rejection over the news I've delivered. For most, there is a stunned silence, then questions about how it happened as they struggle to make sense of the unthinkable.

I marvel at their resiliency. Later, the full force of this loss will strike them heavily as the wife reaches over in bed to touch him gently, or they miss his presence at the dinner table. At this moment, however, I am moved by the human spirit and the ability to maintain a reflective composure in the face of such sudden sadness.

I stay with this family as long as I can, trying to become a part of their unique process. Oddly enough, despite their tragedy, I feel energized. Their brave responses remind me of the courage that is often needed to contend with the unpredictable wonder of living.

Why Bother?

 ON A WARM AND SUNNY AFTERNOON in late May, the streets of Santa Fe were alive with cars cruising and young people gathered on corners and at private parties. It was graduation day at the two local high schools—a day of joy and celebration. But one young man, for reasons unclear and perhaps never understood, took a different path that afternoon.

The call came in to 911. Shouts were heard in the background as the caller said frantically, "Someone has been shot. My God, come quickly!"

The fire department dispatched an ambulance unit with two paramedics on board while a paramedic lieutenant sped off in his rescue truck. As they rushed with lights and sirens through the crowded town, little conversation passed between the two men. Both felt a familiar sick and tight feeling deep inside, for these were the emergency calls they hated the most. Not only was a shooting a difficult case to handle, but the paramedics themselves could be at risk, since the violence might still be rampant. The presence of police assistance could not be assured, at least in the first few moments.

They arrived at the southside house, which stood on dusty ground above an arroyo. Twenty to thirty pickup trucks and lowrider cars were parked haphazardly around a new single-story dwelling. Teenagers gathered in a cluster motioned the ambulance to a pickup parked near the back of the house.

Cautiously, they opened the door to find a young man cradled in the arms of a teenage girl who was quietly sobbing. He was seventeen years old and lived in a small village twenty-five miles away. It was one of the dozens of hamlets that dot the mountainsides of northern New Mexico where generation after generation of Hispanic families have eked out an existence for hundreds of years. Educational stimuli were low; jobs were nonexistent; frustrations ran high.

He had attended a graduation party at the southside house, but during the festivities something had gone terribly wrong. Perhaps too much alcohol, or an argument with his girlfriend, or long-smoldering despair from having grown up in a poor village offering few options— no one was sure. Struck with a sudden madness, he had gone to his pickup truck, pulled a pistol from beneath the seat, placed it to his left temple, and fired.

By the time the paramedics arrived, he was unconscious, appearing asleep in his young friend's arms. After feeling for a carotid pulse, to no avail, they quickly removed him from the truck and began administering CPR, pumping his chest, all the while forcing air into his lungs through a mask.

His injuries seemed minimal—a small entrance wound in the scalp, with some matted, bloody hair surrounding it. Yet his otherwise peaceful appearance, as the paramedics knew all too well, was a facade hiding the catastrophe he had sustained.

Another ambulance arrived with a second crew that furiously began resuscitating the young man. An airway tube was passed into his lungs, and amid the oxygen and forced ventilations, he soon converted from having no pulse to showing a weak but perceptible glimmer of heart activity. A portable heart monitor was then attached, confirming what the paramedics' fingers had already sensed from the young man's wrist. The glow of yellow tracing on the monitor gave out a regular beep, suggesting the promise of life.

The crew's time at the scene had been a brief five minutes, and in another two the ambulance was pulling in the back emergency entrance to the hospital. The young man, now with an intravenous line in his arm, was transferred from the ambulance gurney to a stretcher. A flurry of activity surrounded him as the resuscitation begun so expertly in the field was resumed. His pulse rate was 120, and his blood pressure an acceptable 90. Evidently, his young body had responded quickly to the treatment.

The emergency physician oversaw the practiced routine that followed. Blood specimens were drawn, more intravenous lines begun, and the young man's heart rate and blood pressure electronically monitored by machines hanging on the walls. Meanwhile, a respiratory technician stood at the head of the bed and rhythmically forced oxygen-rich air into his lungs.

After a neurological examination, the young man was rushed off for a CAT scan, to assess the extent of brain damage that had occurred. Five minutes later the first series of pictures were generated by computer, and in another five they were developed and put up on the view box in the emergency department. The attending physicians and nurses looked silently at the black-and-white images of brain, skull, and embedded metal.

The CAT scan showed multiple fragments of bullet material throughout the brain. The fragments lit up with a dense, pure whiteness against the grays and off-white tones of living tissue, suggesting that once viable brain substance was now massively disrupted. Very little of the normal architecture of white-and-gray matter was left; moreover, pools of blood filled the spaces where previously dreams were born and smells of piñon fires on cold nights lovingly recorded.

The doctors and nurses had seen such pictures before. The injuries, they knew, were major—too much had been lost.

A paramedic who had worked hard providing early treatment saw the hopelessness in the eyes of those by the view box. Understandably, given the cumulative stress he experienced every day as an EMT, he was heard to grumble, "All that work trying to save somebody who didn't have a chance. Why bother?"

No one could answer. They just looked away, lost in their own thoughts.

Certainly, no one could blame the young medic for his despair and outburst of frustration. No one there was unaccustomed to mobilizing intense efforts resulting in catastrophe. Emergency medicine is filled with such experiences: long cardiac "codes," irreversible trauma injuries, SIDS deaths. When massive expenditures of time, energy, and supplies are used on patients who don't have a chance, rescue efforts often feel like an excessive struggle. Why preserve a life that is all too fragile and fleeting?

But in this case, the distinction between life and death was not clear. And events over the next fourteen hours shed new light on the importance of striving, no matter how frustrating it may be, to preserve the delicate threads of life.

Despite his irreversible brain damage, the young man's other functions were still viable. Because he'd been resuscitated quickly, no damage had occurred to his heart, kidneys, or other organs. Furthermore, his blood pressure was strong now that his breathing was controlled by the respirator. Everything except his brain was still functional.

The neurosurgeon spent long hours with the grieving family while their loved one lay unresponsive in the intensive care unit. "Chances of recovery are nil," he explained. "It is only the machines that are maintaining some semblance of life." After a while he gently posed the difficult question.

Being simple, deeply religious people, they seemed to reach a decision more quickly than would a family from a more complex setting. They agreed to stop the "machines." If nothing could be done to save their son, then perhaps others could benefit from his tragedy, they reasoned. They agreed to allow his organs to be used for transplants.

All it took was one phone call to activate the national transplant hotline. Instantly, the message was sent around the country to medical centers that specialize in transplanting organs, and within hours special surgical teams were flying in from Wisconsin and Arizona to the small local airport, with surgical instruments and transport cases in hand.

By 6:00 A.M., the local hospital's operating room was prepared. Following strict protocols, the young man's life support machinery was turned off so that his vital signs would cease before the harvesting of organs took place. Then three teams of surgeons expertly removed the young man's heart, pancreas, and both kidneys; it was over in less than thirty minutes.

No sooner were the organs placed in cooled containers than the surgical teams, bearing their precious gifts, were rushed back to the airport in the same ambulance that had brought the young man to the hospital eight hours before. As the sun was rising over the eastern mountains, small jets sped off carrying three of the organs to Minneapolis and Tucson; a separate ground ambulance transported the remaining kidney to Albuquerque. Time was of the essence to get the organs into needy recipients.

Here is a tally of the young man's contribution to others:

• Heart—successfully transplanted in a thirty-nine-year-old Tucson father of a two-year-old. Patient doing well.

• Pancreas—transplanted in a thirty-nine-year-old woman from rural Minnesota with severe diabetes. Currently, she is in remission and may never need insulin again.

• Right kidney—transplanted in a twenty-two-year-old doctoral student from Minneapolis who is now back in classes and doing well.

• Left kidney—transplanted in a sixty-two-year-old man from Albuquerque who had been on chronic dialysis. Patient doing well.

Although nothing could possibly justify the tragic death of a seventeen year old with a full life ahead of him, in this instance it allowed four people to get a new lease on life. Following the meaninglessness of the young man's sudden act, there evolved renewed purpose in the acts of others. Through his death there arose an opportunity for new life.

"Why bother?" he had asked. A question that is echoed repeatedly as technological advances continue to prolong life past the point at which it can be appreciated. Yet for the paramedics, nurses, and doctors who worked so relentlessly to preserve life amid clear indications that it was not to be, the final chapter in this recurring story gave some answers. The conclusion, they all agreed on that summer day, is that the essence of life is a precious entity well worth fighting for.

Little White Crosses

DRIVE DOWN ANY WIDE-OPEN HIGHWAY in the Southwest, especially in the borderlands of Indian country, and you'll see them. Little white crosses. Knee-high, plain wooden crosses standing a few yards off the asphalt, their whiteness in stark contrast to the browns of desert grass and tumbleweed. Solitary and far from civilization, the crosses are often surrounded by neat bouquets of bright plastic flowers. They stand alone, braced against the wind and time.

Each cross marks a special location, the place where someone experienced a violent death from trauma—that severe and sudden bodily injury that remains New Mexico's major health problem. An automobile crash, a pedestrian struck without warning . . . the results are all the same. Placed in loving memory by a family member, typically either Indian or Hispanic, the crosses are left there not only to commemorate the spot but, more importantly, to neutralize the "evil" energy of the event. To the native peoples of those areas, such attempts to restore the balance by countering evil with goodness are important to maintaining health in everyone.

Could it be that trauma actually does have evil or "bad" energy? Are those crosses the humble symbols of unsophisticated people or is

135

there more? Could it be that sudden, catastrophic traumatic events have their own negative karma?

Trauma—from the Greek *traumatikos*, meaning "wound." We in New Mexico who work on any level of EMS are far from novices when it comes to trauma. We live it. Trauma is the name of the game for most of us, from field personnel to the surgeons and critical-care nurses in hospitals. New Mexico holds the notorious distinction of leading the nation every year in death rates from motor vehicle crashes, and is often second in all trauma deaths.

But New Mexico holds no monopoly on trauma. From the often mean inner-city streets of New York to the rain-drenched Cascade Mountains of the Northwest, trauma faces everyone, all the time.

Trauma is our driving force in EMS. Both its incidence and the energy we put into fighting off the deluge of its seemingly endless calls do much to fuel our systems, enhance our training, buy our equipment, even pay our bills.

But is there anyone among us who does not hold lingering images of horrible trauma, images that return to us in dream states or shake us to the core when we hear the wail of sirens or the beep-beep-beep of our pagers?

For me, it was the man who attempted suicide with a rifle pressed under his chin, who only partially succeeded but removed most of his face in the process. For others, there are bold, disturbing memories of deformed or severed limbs, of faces bloodied and swollen beyond recognition. For those of us with many years in EMS under our belts, the images seem at times so frequent that they blur and become generalized. They are the stuff of nightmares.

What is it about the essence of trauma that could be considered "bad"? The events are frequently violent and wrenching. They happen suddenly, often without warning, and forever change the person's experience and the lives of those close to them. There is blood and pain and screaming from the core of the soul. Being in the midst of dealing with a severe trauma case feels at times like being within a circle in Dante's *Inferno*.

Has anyone ever said to you, upon learning that you work in emergency medicine, "Boy, I don't know how you do it—I could never deal with all the things you see"? It's been heard by every EMT, nurse, and emergency physician. Typically, I slough it off; but after fighting for hours to keep alive a trauma victim who is struggling, wailing, and bleeding from wounds too numerous to count, I sense the place from which it comes.

Trauma also holds strong ambivalence. For as much as its bad karma is draining, there is an excitement to it as well. There are those who say they "love" the trauma. Are they crazy? I think not.

Trauma care is palpable. You can get your hands on it and into it; you can see the body's insult and do something about it. It's not like abdominal pain or shortness of breath—especially out in the field, where it's difficult for an EMT to discern what's going on and the available treatment possibilities are minimal.

Trauma care is real. There is an excitement in the doing of it. Results can be quickly seen. It's immediate and straightforward and blood-red. It strikes you in the face, and its sights and sounds reverberate through your being.

The draining energy of trauma care typically does not affect us while we're on the scene. In the critical phase, there is too much to be done. The patient's survival depends on us being clear and functional—for we are the best chance they have at that passionate moment.

But later, in the quiet time, when the patient has been delivered to the hospital and wheeled off to surgery or the intensive care unit or the morgue—the uncomfortable energy begins to show itself. Images creep back, and disturbing memories are recorded in that deep place in the brain where such things reside.

We have much stress in the world of EMS. There are long hours and uncertainties and sometimes even personal danger. But the negative and enervating spirit of trauma has its own special place in that stress milieu.

And it will revisit us again and again. Trauma will not go away, despite our heartfelt efforts to identify its causes and find positive ways of preventing the carnage. For us in EMS, trauma seems destined to remain not only our lifeblood but also the stuff of our nightmares. I am reminded of both each time I drive by a little white cross.

Little Black Boxes

I HAD A DREAM THE OTHER NIGHT. The dream took place in the dim light of future days. Streets were filled with masses of people, mostly old and frail, walking about aimlessly. All had little black boxes about the size of a pager on their hips. Suddenly a man collapsed to the ground. The little black device began to glow, administering an electrical jolt, whereupon he arose to continue his wanderings.

I awoke in a sweat. Was it a nightmare?

A bit far-fetched you might say—but after all, that's what dreams are. To me, the dream symbolizes a growing situation in the world of emergency medicine that eventually will touch us all.

The hottest items on the EMS frontier are defibrillators, both automatic and semiautomatic—electronic devices to counteract the sudden, irregular heartbeats that can be fatal to patients. EMS services throughout New Mexico are acquiring these devices. Advertisements for the "little boxes" fill EMS journals. There is tremendous vendor pressure to market the devices even before systems are ready to accommodate them. My agency, for example, was recently contacted by a public swimming pool manager in a northern New Mexico community that had purchased an automatic defibrillator and was wondering what to do with it.

This technology is rapidly expanding. High-risk heart patients are often sent home from the hospital with automatic defibrillators, and their families instructed in its use. There is a prototype of a cardiac rhythm device for home use, tied in by telemetry to the hospital intensive care unit and designed to "shock" over the airways should a critical rhythm develop. Feeling a little puny today? Just plug in your defibrillator. Forget about those heart troubles . . . Carry your little black box around. It's the millennial version of the "forever young" mindset—except it goes one step further, by offering the subtle promise of immortality as well.

I view widespread availability of automatic defibrillators as a major symbolic leap in the world of EMS, and one that could provide a longer life expectancy, freedom from suffering, and pleasure in the moment. But at what cost?

The technology that most dramatically illuminates this trade-off is nuclear energy. That promise of an unending power source is countered by the horrible possibility of making the planet uninhabitable for future generations. I don't want to imply that an automatic defibrillator in your local restaurant and on every street corner is as complex an issue as nuclear weapons and meltdowns at Chernobyl. Still there is a factor in the widespread acceptance of automatic defibrillators that causes concern.

The implied promise is that if we can recognize a critical heart arrhythmia and shock it quickly enough, the patient will be saved and go on to experience the many pleasures of life. With this false promise comes a public expectation that emergency providers can accomplish anything—that all EMTs, doctors, and nurses, if given the right "tools," can reverse any human condition that brings death and suffering. Heart stopped? Give it a shock. Coronary artery clogged? Give it a new high-tech drug like tPa—an overly priced Drano brewed from vats of mutant bacteria—and dissolve that clot. Got a kidney stone? Let's blast it into the cosmos with some ultra-ultrasound.

The truth is that we cannot do everything. We cannot reverse most sudden death or the natural course of aging. And with the spread of slick devices like defibrillators, those of us who practice medicine may be pressured into accepting the lie that we can save everyone— even those at the very end of the natural and inevitable journey known as the human experience.

I have seen it in the faces of paramedics. I have felt it too often myself. We become frustrated after spending hours trying to resuscitate someone in ventricular fibrillation. We have given all the right drugs; we have shocked repeatedly on what should be a reversible condition; and still we can't change the inevitable.

The lie that we can do everything is one we desperately wish were true, for in large measure, we are in the field of EMS to save lives and alleviate suffering. It is what we do. It is our purpose.

For that reason I don't propose to ban the defibrillator. It is a potentially important device capable of saving lives in certain situations and should therefore be a part of our bag of tools. But how can we slow this rush toward uncontrolled technology so that automatic defibrillators are not advertised in Sears catalogs or wired up to the pay phone in your corner restaurant?

As the "experts" in emergency care, we must educate the public, institutions, and government agencies about what all this new technology means. There are appropriate uses of almost any device, as long as it takes its proper place as just one part of the EMS system, and not an isolated contraption promising resurrection and eternal life.

We need to spend a measure of time asking more metaphysical, philosophical questions about the promises and expectations we give to the public and ourselves. What can we realistically provide? Ongoing discussion of living wills, Do Not Resuscitate orders, and quality of life for all members of society. All the while, we need to question what technological advances do—and don't do—for the world.

There are no ready answers to these difficult ethical questions, but in the asking, answers eventually may come. And then the "little black boxes" may become our allies rather than our rulers.

Fiery Wreck

EVER SINCE READING THE NEWSPAPER ACCOUNT, I'd been interested to see the spot where the accident occurred. The article was quite short, more a news brief than a real story, which surprised me, given the visceral content of the tragic event.

On Interstate 25, almost midway between Santa Fe and Albuquerque, on a bright afternoon with normal weather conditions, a pickup truck with California tags was traveling north at what witnesses stated was a high rate of speed. It suddenly veered across the median, crossed into the southbound lanes, and collided cataclysmically with a truck from another state. Both vehicles immediately burst into flames, preventing any attempt to get to the victims. The newspaper piece ended by matter-of-factly stating that neither driver had yet been identified, since rescuers could find only charred skeletons in the tangled mass of metal.

A few days later, on my next trip to Albuquerque, I tried to see where it happened. Close to the exit for Santo Domingo Pueblo, I came upon it. The knee-high grass in the median was trampled in a linear swath, as if some giant eraser had passed over it. The small chain-link fence separating the two sides of the interstate now sport-ed a gaping ten-foot hole. And there on the southbound lanes was a thirty-foot circular patch of blackened and oily residue, which would discolor the grayish asphalt for years to come.

As I drove directly through the black stain at sixty-five miles per hour, I felt a palpable shiver come over me. Something deep inside sensed the moment of screeching tires, twisted metal, and sudden evaporation of two lives.

Just another day on New Mexico highways. Anyone involved with EMS and emergency care in our state has an intimate relationship with the trauma on our roads and in our communities. We continue to lead the nation in mortality figures for vehicular deaths, and are right near the top for trauma of all kinds. It is our constant companion.

No wonder so many people keep working to develop a better system of trauma care for our state. No sophisticated system would have reversed the fire on I-25 that day (except perhaps prevention), but what if the scenario had been a bit different?

What if the wreck had not been so intensely final, and if the two victims, although severely injured, had not died? With rapid access to 911 through a passing motorist's cellular phone, the first response could be swift and effective. Standardized triage and transport protocols could be in place with the local EMS service, and the Lifeguard helicopter accessed immediately. The designated trauma center in Albuquerque would then go on alert. The victims would be quickly stabilized by various levels of providers at the scene, all of whom were trained in prehospital life support. Then the patients would be evacuated by air to the hospital, through the emergency department, into the operating room, and finally into intensive care. Despite their critical injuries, the victims might well recuperate. And by tracking data on them through the system of prehospital, hospital, and rehabilitative care, emergency personnel might learn more about the preventive and acute-care aspects of trauma that could make a difference in the next such event.

Trauma system development is, I've become acutely aware, a long and sometimes arduous process. There are countless meetings, endless drafts of regulations, and tough negotiations with all the players in trauma care, as we try to reach consensus. At times, I wonder if all the effort is worth it.

But then I drive over densely stained spots on the highway where reality comes rushing back and screams in my face. When I do, this effort, it seems, is certainly worthwhile. Not only worthwhile, but desperately needed.

Field of Dreams

 IN A 1995 ISSUE of the nationally known trade journal
JEMS was an article about the hottest topic in emergency
medical services around the country: the expanded-scope
practice of EMTs. The story centered on the Sand Key II Conference
in Florida, where movers and shakers met to again discuss the progress
of expanded EMS on many fronts.

The reports out of Sand Key II were not nearly as optimistic as the
brave new world envisioned at the Sand Key I convened back in 1994,
when this topic was first openly discussed. In the year and a half that passed
between the two Florida-based gatherings, there evolved a series of political, legal, and financial realities that effectively grounded the grandiose
plans of both urban and rural expanded-EMS projects all over the country. Virtually every system where expanded EMS was contemplated—
including the former flagship program in Pinellas County, Florida—was
now as dead in the water as a yacht with a blown engine in Tampa Bay.

Except one such program. The article in *JEMS* stated it clearly:
"The only folks ready to tell [of their successes] were the people from
tiny Red River, New Mexico—the only place in the United States
where paramedics have actually learned a full range of new skills and
are officially providing treatment to patients they don't transport."

In September 1996, I went to Red River for an emotional two-day gathering to put the final touches on that community's groundbreaking experience in expanded EMS. The three-year federal demonstration grant that launched this unique program was ending, and a handful of us involved since its inception had come together for an official close-out evaluation—to look hard at its successes, its failures, and the lessons learned from it.

Red River is magical in autumn, which comes early to northern New Mexico's high elevations. The aspens turn yellow on the mountainsides, frost appears on car windows each morning, and tourists stop dreaming about twenty-inch trout and start dreaming of ski slopes with twenty inches of fresh powder.

I awoke early in the morning and walked the almost deserted main street of the village. Mist was rising off the rushing river, and the sweet smell of smoke from newly stocked woodstoves hung in the air. Red River seemed such a simple and untouched place—not at all like the glorified center of expanded EMS for the entire nation.

Our nine-member evaluation group met in the firehouse's second-story conference room. The large bare room was where much of the expanded paramedic training initially took place. Some anatomical charts graced the walls, and an old bookshelf in the corner was filled with medical texts. Just off the training room, Red River EMS had set up its makeshift "clinic," staffed by expanded-practice medic Ron Burnham and his colleagues. There on a daily basis they handled manageable emergencies such as simple wounds and earaches, so that residents of the isolated and doctorless community would not have to travel the forty-five tough miles through mountain passes to the closest hospital emergency room.

As the nine of us sat around a conference table the first morning, people from the village steadily passed by to visit with the "new doc" next door. Some paused to say hello, to talk about the weather—and perhaps to suspiciously wonder about all these strangers hanging out at the fire station.

Our official evaluation group did its duty. We looked at the entire demonstration project's goals, its accomplishments, its failings. We looked toward the future, to determine how the lessons learned in Red River might help other communities—not only in this state, but on a broader national plane as well. We were thorough and conscientious in our deliberations.

But despite our serious task, I couldn't help feeling we were like children opening presents on a holiday morning. It was a celebration— of having watched and nurtured this infant of an idea as it grew into a breathing, functional entity that people around the nation would point to as a model for the future of EMS.

During those days in the fire station, my mind wandered back to images from the previous four years:

• The original consortium of folks from Red River, Taos, the local hospital and medical community, the EMS Academy, the EMS Bureau, and others who brainstormed the concept in preparation for submitting the original grant application;

• The frequent meetings—often accentuated by heated debates—with local physicians and hospital staff, about whether this plan was intended to improve health care for people in the area or to sound the first death knell for American medicine as we knew it;

• The endless drafts of curriculum and treatment protocols developed by the EMS Academy, local physicians, and the EMS Bureau staff as we tried to define this new provider;

• The long hours of didactic and clinical training endured by that local cadre of paramedics as they challenged themselves to extend their vision beyond their traditional roles;

• The flood of requests for information from EMS services around the county, and all the invitations to speak at national conferences, from people hungry to learn what took place in Red River;

• Attending general sessions and workshops on the project at the annual State EMS Conference in July and, best of all, watching with pride as Ron Burnham and Dr. Alfredo Vigil of Red River were given special awards for their long hours of dedication to emergency medicine and to the concept of expanded EMS.

The Red River experiment—aptly renamed the New Mexico Project—stimulated such interest that the legislature was petitioned in 1996 to consider extending the program throughout the state. Lawmakers were asked to tackle the legal and financial hurdles so that other New Mexico communities, where appropriate, could tap into expanded EMS as a partial answer to the statewide health-care crisis.

And the legislature responded by passing Senate Joint Memorial #44, which directed the state Department of Health to convene a broad-based committee to explore the entire process and make suggestions on its implications throughout New Mexico. Led by the EMS Bureau, the committee immediately went to work on a report. Its recommendations should set the course of expanded EMS for years to come.

During the lunchtime break on our first day of evaluations, our group made its way from the firehouse to a nearby eatery on Red River's main street. I found myself walking a few paces behind Ron Burnham and other expanded-practice medics who serve as the new health providers in town. Local residents passed by in old pickup trucks, honking their horns, waving, and calling out hellos. People on the street stopped to share a bit of gossip and let the medics know how "Grandma" was doing with her new blood-pressure medicine. The pace of little Red River slowed considerably for these known and trusted providers of health care as they walked down the street to get some lunch.

Maybe it was the altitude depriving my brain of needed oxygen, but at that moment I was overwhelmed by the "rightness" of the scene in downtown Red River. The feeling was not specifically linked to Ron Burnham and his colleagues, or to the picturesque village surrounding us, or even to the honesty of rural communities in general. No, it had to do with what the health of people is all about. It was a longing for simpler times, when "health care" meant chancing upon your doctor on the street and having time to talk about the weather.

In the now-classic 1989 film *Field of Dreams*, based on a W. P. Kinsella novel, a simple Iowa farmer keeps hearing voices telling him to build a baseball diamond in the middle of his cornfield. "Build it and he will come . . ." the voice keeps imploring. Well, here in Red

River, New Mexico, we have built it and they come. From around the nation, and even beyond our borders, people involved with EMS are writing, calling, and even visiting to learn more about this grand experiment, this field of dreams.

Like most dreams, the hopes and realities at times get a bit muddled, and everything we hope for doesn't always come to pass. But in the village of Red River on that cool September morning, what had happened seemed just right to me, and a source of pride to all the people in New Mexico.

Part Three

GATHERING SHADOWS

(December 1993–December 1998)

*A*t the age of forty-eight, I was discovered to have
the recurrence of a rare and nasty malignancy that
first appeared when I was twenty-two. For the next five
years, I was locked into cycles of remissions, exacerbations,
and a world turned upside down. Between multiple
surgeries and radiation treatments, I worked as an assistant
professor at the New Mexico School of Medicine and
served as the medical director of the state's Emergency
Medical Services Bureau. But my core involvement was
as "the doctor as a fragile patient" facing a progressive
deadly adversary. Lessons learned from Indian people
and complementary healing provided the best spiritual
medicine in coming to peace with the cycles of time and
helped me contend with the depression I often felt in letting go of my deep connections with this life.

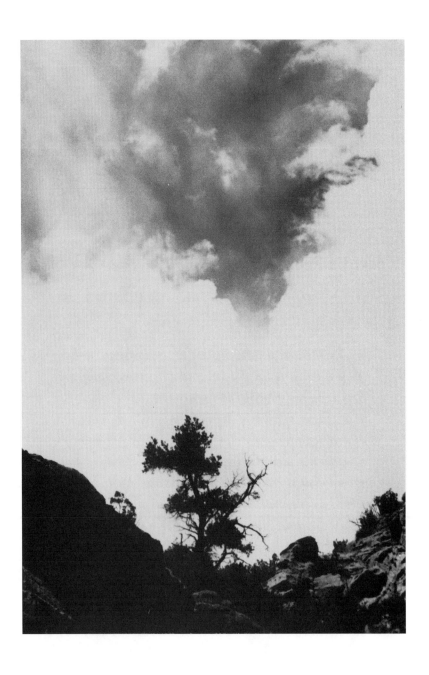

When the Doctor Gets Sick

IT ALL BEGAN INNOCUOUSLY ENOUGH one Saturday afternoon while I was working at the hospital. The emergency department shift had been busy, for the late spring day had suddenly exploded with the warmth of midsummer, and everyone was out and about, running into one another, tripping and spraining and doing those deeds that eventually bring them to the hospital.

About 4:00 P.M., I began having chills, malaise, and muscle aches. Between seeing patients, I stuck a thermometer in my mouth and found my temperature to be 102°. Not thinking much about it (in that setting we're frequently hit with a variety of strange viruses), I threw down two aspirins and shivered through the last five hours of my shift.

All night at home I continued to chill and ache; even sleep was fitful and fleeting. The next day the fever continued, almost 105° at times, despite a steady intake of aspirin that made my ears ring and stomach complain. That night I broke into a profuse sweat, whereupon the fever broke.

The following day I was listless and wasted, which seemed consistent with overcoming a virus that had run its course. The event was over and I went about my business. Little did I know that the next month and a half would dispel any notion that this was a simple infection quickly contracted, quickly overcome.

Six days later the fever returned, with a temperature of 105° and shaking chills. It again lasted two days and then mysteriously disappeared, with a crisis of sweats as I soaked through five T-shirts during the night. The second day of the fever I had to work a twelve-hour shift at the hospital; and although it was at times painful, with some aspirin and forced avoidance of concern the long day was put behind me.

Before leaving that evening, I went to the hospital lab for a blood test to see what might be happening. I also ran into a friend—an internist and specialist in infectious diseases—as he was finishing his late rounds. He was nice enough to examine me in his office.

My blood count was equivocal. The white cell count (a loose indicator of infection) was not elevated, and the types of cells suggested a viral illness. But surprisingly and most troublesome, the level of red cells was significantly depressed, to a point where I was down about three units of blood.

My friend checked me over well, but couldn't find an obvious source of infection such as pneumonia, strep throat, or bubonic plague—something we in New Mexico are always alert to. Nevertheless, he started me on antibiotics, and I went home to sweat again. The next morning I returned to the lab for a complete series of blood tests, which all looked fairly normal in liver function, kidney status, and general metabolism.

After the fever, I again felt fatigued and weak. Over the next five days, however, my temperature remained stable, so I figured I had turned the corner. But then, as if some internal clock were ticking, the high fevers began anew. Another blood count showed significant anemia, worse than before.

By this time, the relapsing fevers were taking their toll both physically and spiritually. I had lost about ten pounds, which on my slender frame was easily noticeable. My regular jogging and bicycling were out of the question; even the slightest exertion left me breathless.

But more importantly, I was beginning to feel an unrelenting uneasiness with the disharmony my body was experiencing. As a physician, I knew enough about disease to realize that this might not be just a simple infective process, but something more serious, more insidious.

When a doctor is faced with a patient who has relapsing fevers, anemia, and no focus of infection, the differential diagnosis quickly begins to include a litany of frightening entities: lymphoma, leukemia, Hodgkin's disease, renal tumors, or a primary cancer that has not yet shown itself but has invaded the bone marrow.

The next weeks were not easy. I awoke each morning with a fear of finding a new symptom, a new setback. I'd check for enlarged glands in my neck, for a tender spleen, for weight loss. Waiting for the final diagnosis became an obsession. I lived each day with a growing undercurrent of anxiety. Through it all, I continued to work and attempt fairly normal relationships at home. In retrospect, however, I was unable to keep up the masquerade on either front.

Four weeks after the first chills, the fever returned, lasting two days and then mysteriously disappearing as before. I had another physical exam and another series of blood tests. Still no conclusive evidence of either an infective process or a malignancy, just the anemia. My doctor thought my prostate gland seemed a bit enlarged, and although I didn't fit the picture of prostatitis by either urine or blood tests, he put me on a powerful (and expensive) antibiotic considered the best for chronic prostatitis.

Whatever the reason—the antibiotics, a viral infection that had just run its course, or a combination of the two—the fevers did not return. The first time I passed the mystical period of six to seven days with no symptoms, I was surprised yet wary. More blood was drawn. It still showed the anemia, although with slight improvement.

Then my strength began to return. I remember one important day when I walked a brisk two miles with minimal breathlessness near my home north of Santa Fe. My apprehension was beginning to fade.

But another psychological setback was in the cards. In the first phase of my illness, then again three weeks later, I'd had blood samples sent to the state laboratory for special serum examinations called "acute" and "convalescent." Often, this is the only way to discover the cause of a bizarre infective process, since if the two specimens show a change in certain antibodies to viruses or bacteria, the agent responsible for the infection can be identified. I saw this as a definitive test, for if it traced my symptoms to a Coxsackie virus or rickettsia parasite, such as the tick whose bite causes Rocky Mountain spotted fever, then the chances of an occult malignancy would be null and void.

The pathologist called when he received the results. The information, however, was more like a nonresult. The lab had been unable to successfully check any of my specimens for antibody levels, because some unknown and rare substance in my blood prevented completion of the test. "What could that substance be?" I asked. The list included four or five possibilities, all fairly bizarre. But as a final suggestion, the pathologist voiced a concern about Hodgkin's disease, a type of cancer that attacks the lymph nodes.

This last test result again draped a shroud of uncertainty over my life. Yet each day passed without fever, with an improvement in my blood counts, and with a gradual return of weight and strength, convincing me that my mysterious affliction had finally come to an end. Soon I was able to stop the obsessive concerns and get on with living. The illness, I figured, was history—just another piece of the puzzle that makes our lives so intense at times.

Maybe it really was prostatitis or a viral infection, although I suspect it was actually a tick-borne relapsing fever that was not detected on the initial blood tests. I remember that about ten days before the first onset of fever I was bitten by an unseen insect while putting on my jeans one morning at a campsite in a place called Chaco Canyon—a mystical, powerful site of ancestral Indian ruins in northwestern New Mexico, and to me and my family an important spiritual center. How ironic that Chaco Canyon might have been at the source of those six weeks of uncertainty, fear, and glimpses of mortality!

So it ended, and life went on. Although in the midst of the turmoil there were frightening moments, in retrospect the illness and my response to it were simple. As a doctor would put it, I'd had an infective process that ran its course without any lingering sequelae. In my world of emergency medicine, I see more devastating and irreversible tragedies every day. My illness was easy compared with the events affecting so many others—the loss of a loved one, discovery of cancer in a teenager, sudden death in an automobile crash.

Even so, important lessons were learned through that experience. The most memorable one was a crash course in how doctors face the uncertainty of sickness in themselves.

Physicians try to put themselves above constant reflections on mortality, vulnerability, and dependency. Perhaps as a protective mechanism, the doctor tends not to burden himself with such considerations when the patients he treats are faced with major illness. But when the doctor get sick, those protective walls crumble. Intimations of one's own mortality become paralyzing and terrifying.

The first illusion to go is that of the doctor's omnipotence. In treating most illnesses, we feel that our powers of intellect and deduction, coupled with the "magic bullets" of antibiotics and drugs at our disposal, can overwhelm even the most elusive pathogens. Such an assumption is understandable, since modern medicine does have a record of success with most ailments—although its ability to deal with the complex interplay of body, mind, spirit, and environment leaves much to be desired.

For me the powers were suddenly gone. Not only did this illness not play by the rules, but everything we tried at the onset was ineffective.

My core was also shaken by a newly discovered sense of vulnerability. Doctors don't get sick—it's always the others, the patients, who come down with illnesses. When the roles were reversed and it was I who was fragile and dependent, the fear of vulnerability was perhaps a greater load on my psyche than the fear of finding an enlarged lymph node in the neck.

Because the unfamiliar feelings of powerlessness, vulnerability, and dependency were so draining, I found myself denying that any serious problem could actually be taking place. That, coupled with the arrogance of thinking I knew everything about disease processes, caused me to enter into self-diagnosis and self-treatment. It quickly becomes a slippery slide, this business of the doctor treating himself, and one that can all too often lead to addiction and substance abuse among health professionals.

I also found myself "chasing numbers" from all my lab tests and daily weight checks. Rather than simply asking myself, "How do you feel today?" I became obsessed with the degree of my anemia. Was the hemoglobin level up 0.5 grams in the past week, which was to be expected? Was my bone marrow production depressed to 15 percent of normal? These scientific intellectual exercises got in the way of relating to the more important considerations of how my body and spirit were feeling at those particular moments. It was only after I refused to undergo any more blood tests that my feelings of strength and optimism began to rebound. Ignorance was certainly bliss.

It was about this time, when I had emotionally rejected the scientific approach to my illness, that I began seriously considering non-medical treatments. I had long been an advocate of restoring harmony by elevating the importance of spirit and environment—the holistic approach to treating illness. Now was my chance to practice what had been mostly an intellectual joust in the past, and to utilize the power of my own self to battle this fever.

I began forcing a full and nutritious diet on myself, even when I was not hungry. I took megadosages of vitamins, especially vitamin C. I set aside time for meditating and playing with imagery and taking long walks. I spent as much time as possible in the mountains, hiking along streams as they rushed out of isolated canyons and watching flickers work tree bark for food.

I went fishing, although I secretly hoped not to catch anything; life of any sort was too precious to take. And I spent every free moment with my two kids. Their joyous abandon in play was infectious and healing.

I reread Norman Cousins's *Anatomy of an Illness*, which chronicles his bout with a debilitating and untreatable disease he contracted in

1964. Faced with this painful illness, for which the medicines he was taking were more destructive than the pathological process itself, Cousins began an organized approach to self-healing through laughter and good thoughts.

He had friends bring old Marx Brothers movies to his hospital room, where he would watch them by the hour and notice how laughter and smiles lessened the pain and stimulated recovery. I took the 1980s approach to his prescription by raiding every video store in town and watching hours of Monty Python and Mel Brooks cinemas.

Every little bit helped: the concern and care of a sensitive doctor who worked with me through the frustrations, the warmth of my family, the vitamins, the long walks, the funny movies. All contributed to my eventual recovery.

Now, as I work with patients who come to the hospital, no matter how minor their complaints may be I find myself remembering the lessons learned during those six weeks—the fear and helplessness, the vulnerability and concern that maybe, just maybe, something really serious is going on. Those fears are counterproductive to the healing process, for illness feeds on hopelessness and succumbs to optimism.

For every setback I experienced during those intense weeks, I gained a twofold insight into the human condition and how we respond to illness. And I developed a lasting appreciation of the sometimes delicate and fragile plain we all walk upon, where a little fever, a little chill, can shake important foundations.

My New Life
As a Patient

AT FORTY-EIGHT YEARS OLD, I'm having a bout with a nasty tumor in my neck. By all accounts, it's a reemergence almost twenty-six years after it first appeared. That seems a long time for a tumor to take to return and, to my thinking, represents a cosmic joke in which I've yet to see the humor. Although there are clear physical distinctions between this occurrence and the first, the most palpable contrast I feel is how differently I handled the news when I was a twenty-two year old, full of life and possibilities, and how I am handling it now in midlife.

It was summer, back in the tumultuous '60s, and I was about to start medical school when I noticed a relatively painless lump on the left side of my neck. After a few months, when I began losing weight and hypertension kicked in, I decided to have it checked.

I was admitted to our community hospital for a simple biopsy, which showed the lump to be the tip of a substantial mass that extended deep into my neck. I had a tumor of the carotid body, called a chemodectoma. Typically slow-growing and uncommonly malignant, though locally invasive, it fell into a strange class of glomus tumors that earn the classification "rare." So my care was put in the hands of a vascular specialist at the university I was about to attend.

I began medical school in September. And as I struggle to remember that time in 1967, I cannot recall being especially worried or unable to keep my mind on my studies. I was young, enrolled in a prestigious medical school, and my future felt rosy to the core. Not only that, but I had great trust in modern medicine. In my smartly starched white coat, I was just discovering its wonders.

Over Christmas break that first semester, I checked into the hospital and, without asking many questions, lay down on the operating table for what turned out to be eight hours of surgery. In order to fully remove the nasty neoplasm, the surgeons who operated on me had to sacrifice a number of other useful pieces of my anatomy, such as cranial nerves and carotid arteries. But the good news was that the tumor was gone.

I recuperated quickly and was soon back in classes. I was left with some impairment—only one usable vocal cord, for instance—but it was damage I've mostly been able to hide, even from the most observant of my fellow physicians.

I went on to finish medical school, take an old-fashioned rotating internship, join the US Public Health Service, and settle in the Southwest, working with Indian tribes and doing an occasional emergency room shift at the local hospital. Eventually, I become board certified in emergency medicine and the medical director of a busy Level II trauma center.

Along the way, I married, had two children, and developed a full and busy life. Jogging, skiing, and indulging in other vigorous pastimes were not precluded by the long-forgotten surgery. The tumor was past history.

Fast forward to 1994.

We deny so much, especially as the subtle aches and pains of age begin creeping in. I realized for six months I had been feeling more and more pain on the left side of my neck and occasional dizziness when I moved my head suddenly. But at first it seemed like nothing that the stress of emergency medicine and some pesky slipped cervical disks from an old softball injury couldn't account for. I am not immune to that delusion harbored by doctors, more so than the population at large, that we cannot get sick. But finally, my well-honed denial crumpled. I had developed a firm lymph node on the left side of my neck, and my hearing on that side had noticeably diminished.

I consulted my family practitioner and friend, who was likewise concerned, and checked with another colleague, a radiologist. I soon found myself, shivering and uncomfortable, lying in the surrealistic space-age magnetic chamber of a magnetic resonance imaging (MRI) device. I was scared, alone, and in the cold hands of technology.

The next week was an emotional and sleepless blur. I underwent two more MRI tests, blood studies, a biopsy, and consultations with specialists. The tumor of my youth had come back (or perhaps never been fully removed), and it had turned very nasty. It was now metastatic—very rare for an already rare type of tumor. And most troublesome, a tentacle of the mass had worked its way into my skull and brain stem.

I checked into our hospital for six hours on the operating table, during which the surgeons were able to remove all the intracranial material without sacrificing anything important, like pieces of brain stem, spinal nerves, or my vertebral artery. I began recovering quickly and in four days was able to pry myself out of the hospital and return to the healing comforts of home—although two weeks later I developed aseptic meningitis, a relapse that landed me back in the hospital and briefly shook my faith.

Over many weeks of lying in hospital beds, unsure if it was night or day, and trapped in my bed at home with such severe headaches that sitting up was a major effort, I've thought about what it means to be sick and impaired. As I've gotten better, my days have been spent taking long walks, doing simple exercises, reading, and watching funny videos to stimulate my soul.

But so much uncertainty remains. There is still a sizable mass in the left side of my neck that is putting pressure on nerves and has the distinct possibility of metastasizing to skull or lungs. Will it be operable without destroying the few remaining nerves on that side? Can my neck take another brutal invasion?

I am learning what it is like to be a patient, and it's been a sobering and deeply disturbing journey. One has to give up control, stop intellectualizing about the science of it all, and become dependent, graciously accepting the bowl of chicken soup as the gift of healing it is intended to be. I'm finding that the waiting time—for a biopsy report, for an opening in the surgical schedule—is frightening as hell. Although I know that pessimism is an enemy, optimism is harder to come by. One doesn't just take two pills in the morning to get the faith levels elevated. Positive energy is fragile, I've discovered, fleeing quickly in the face of pain.

In the years since medical school, I have lost my comforting trust in Western medicine. It has its magic bullets and life-saving machines, its dedicated physicians, nurses, and technicians who go the distance for their patients, but I know by now that it can't do everything.

From the Native Americans I have worked with over the years, I've learned to view healing as a restoration of balance between the body, the spirit, and the environment. The sense that there is something larger and more important in the cosmos gives a necessary balance to my immediate and trivial fretting. The friends who have come to visit seem as effective in my healing as the steroids and antibiotics. Counting my blessings has taken on new significance.

Over the course of these months, I have frequently traveled to a spiritual place on Indian Pueblo land near my home, where the sky, trees, and ochre-colored mesas fit together in balance. The eagles fly overhead and the wind whispers through the pines. I pray in that place, lying on the cool earth and trying to feel its strength. This part of my healing journey is a gift from the native people, who are as practiced in their traditional medicine art as the surgeons who carefully removed tumor from my brain stem. All are part of the process.

In the months ahead I'll have more CTs and other tests. Eventually, I'll need more surgery on the neck mass, probably by a team of surgeons at some faraway medical center; perhaps even some radiation to slow down any remaining renegade cells. It's likely that both technological medicine and my own faith will make important contributions.

And finally, I will have to learn to live with whatever pain and disability and doubts remain. For now, the real possibilities of death or severe disability stare me full in the face. What have I accomplished in the time I have been blessed with? Is there so much more to do? A persistent voice within me pleads: *Give me just a little more time with my family and friends. Just a little more time.*

Hard Tables

I AM AGAIN LYING ON A COLD, hard treatment table. They've become a familiar setting over the past eleven months, these tables. Despite the frequency of our contact, I've never gotten used to the solid inflexibility of these slabs of plastic, which offer no comfort to the natural curves of my back and hips.

I was discovered to have a recurrence of a bizarre cancer in my neck eleven months ago. The tumor came back twenty-six years after its initial removal—a very long time for any recurrence and especially unusual for this rare kind of cancer. Since it was discovered, I have been through a course characterized by the inevitable ups and downs experienced by cancer patients. Moments of despair have been countered with flights of optimism. There have been periods of unrelenting pain and times when I've felt as strong and vibrant as I've ever been. Throughout it all, there have been cold, hard tables.

I'm far away from my mountain home, in this surreal high-tech chamber at the medical center in Loma Linda, California. Nestled in the rolling foothills of the San Bernardino Valley east of Los Angeles, Loma Linda is an internationally known medical center where patients from around the globe travel for specialized treatments not always available in their local hospitals. I have come to this mecca of high technology to take advantage of the multimillion-dollar proton accelerator encased in fifteen-foot concrete walls three stories below ground level. It is the country's only regularly operated proton treatment facility, where protons, the "magic bullets" of radiation therapy, are sent at the speed of light into precise trajectories to deliver cell-destroying energy to deep tumors without affecting the surrounding tissue.

But all that cutting-edge technology isn't on my mind today. I can think only of how uncomfortable I am on this table. So many tables like this over the months. My mind wanders, breaking through the meditation mantra I'm attempting to silently recite, returning to the countless tables I've been thrown upon.

The image of those tables comes rushing in like a long line of flatbed railroad cars. The six or seven CT scans. The seven magnetic-resonance-imaging studies. The two arteriograms. The two surgical experiences, averaging almost eight hours each. The three X-ray simulations in preparation for radiation treatment. Five weeks of daily conventional radiation therapy. And now, another afternoon experience on a cold table in the proton accelerator. So many tables.

Some have been diagnostic tables. Others have been for treatment. All have been connected, both physically and emotionally, with that high-tech, computer-based, impersonal, and cold side of Western medicine that holds such a dilemma for us. The technology offers the "miracles" we have come to expect of modern medicine, yet lacks the warmth, the touching, and the healing concern of others. There are no comforting hands in those machines, no steaming chicken soup. It's all grayish-white plastic, fluorescent lights, red laser beams on walls, harsh and whining metallic noises—and always, those cold, hard tables.

This table deep underground at Loma Linda is especially unnerving. It's too short for my six-foot-plus height, so my Achilles tendons jut uncomfortably over the edge during the thirty-minute treatment. The table slides into a gigantic plastic-and-metal doughnut that is only a small part of the truck-size gantry in the treatment room, allowing protons to be focused precisely in any area of the body, from any number of angles. It is like being suspended in the center of a monstrous gyroscope that spins in multiple directions at once. The technicians, after making their initial settings on the table and positioning the proton nozzle, retire to a room far removed and complete the treatment using computers and video cameras. The treatment room is cold and harsh, and after those massive lead doors snap shut I am alone with the protons and laser beams.

For my particular tumor, the daily treatment itself takes only two minutes. A high-pitched electric whine begins building to a crescendo as the protons are accelerated from a source a football field's length away, and then focused with magnetic lenses into one of the four treatment rooms. When the protons actually begin spraying through the nozzle at the speed of light and entering my field, a detector goes off, sounding very much like an electronic door chime. It's almost a pleasing sound, soft and bell-like. More importantly, it reminds me something is working there deep at my skull base, blasting through the DNA material of the tumor, rendering the cells incapable of their malignant intent. Almost as soon as the whining and chiming begin, they quickly disappear, the room becomes silent, and the technicians reenter to extricate me from the hard table and the molded mask that holds me tightly in place. As I walk along the deserted hospital corridors away from of the treatment area, it all seems like a dreamworld—entirely disconnected from my fears and indecisions about future days.

The five-week course of conventional radiation treatment I just finished in my hometown of Santa Fe felt different. The table was still hard, but the surroundings were more homelike and the technicians people I recognized and had a history with. The treatment room at the cancer center in our town's only hospital is large and smacks of high-tech, but gives more sense of space and personal warmth. The treatment beam, which spews out X rays (called photons) and electrons (the small weightless particles that orbit atoms), comes from a gigantic C-arm apparatus that rotates 360 degrees around the patient lying on a stationary table. The individualized, molded plastic mask I wore for each treatment was fixed to the table, locking me in place and producing a strange claustrophobia for the ten or so minutes of each daily treatment.

After the five weeks of treatment ended, I took the mask home, and now occasionally glance at it as if it will talk back, answering my questions. It looks like me, that same profile with prominent nose and high cheekbones, but because I had to assume for each treatment an uncomfortable position in which my neck was severely hyperextended, the mask has a horror movie essence to it. It reminds me of the evil villain's profile in *Alien* and its sequels: lizardlike, with a thin, extended neck and long, sloping forehead.

In moments of morbid jesting to relieve the anxiety of facing cancer, I refer to it as my death mask. At other times, I look at it as my mask of life. It depends on the day.

And all the other hard, cold tables. There have been CT scans and MRIs in numerous cities: Santa Fe, Dallas, Loma Linda. When I had my first MRI years ago after a bizarre softball injury that left three cervical disks herniated, lying in that small, elongated magnetic doughnut was deeply troublesome. I am not by nature a claustrophobic person; but there was something profoundly disturbing about being so encased in a plastic coffin with my nose virtually inches from the ceiling and my body immobilized. Any movement other than hurried breathing was impossible. Escape was out of the question.

Since then, I've been through so many imaging studies that the experience has become almost tolerable. The CT scans are easy. They usually go quickly and feel spacious when compared with an MRI. The sounds of a CT going through its computerized X-ray slices of the anatomy are soft, at times pleasant.

MRIs are still difficult, although not as rattling as that first one. The forty-five minutes or so it takes to complete a study, with and without intravenous injection of a contrast agent, seems to drag on beyond the ticking of a clock. Because the sensitivity of imaging requires the patient to remain totally still, there is tension to keep from swallowing, twitching, or even blinking the eyes. The jarring, grinding sound produced when images are received in the computer is inherently disturbing to some deep core of the brain. It is like being in the middle of a hydraulic car-crusher in an urban wrecker yard.

Faced with so many imaging studies on hard tables, I've developed my own functional method of meditation and self-hypnosis that helps me get through the experience. The stereo earphones the technicians usually offer to drown out metallic sounds of the machine are not helpful, for they break through the discipline I need for self-induced relaxation. I have been able to reach another place from that small doughnut hole in which I find myself—not necessarily a place of great tranquillity, but certainly one of more peacefulness.

I sometimes dream—both in sleep and in those altered states that come over me during treatment—that I'm on another hard and cold table. It's in a brightly lit, bare-walled room of tile. No one else is around. The room is utterly silent except for a rhythmic drip of water into a stainless-steel sink. I lie, covered by a white plastic sheet, on a metal table with slightly raised borders and a drain at one end. It is an autopsy table, and I am the subject matter of the day. I watch this image from the dream state, detached from its reality. It is just a place, not an emotion. It is final.

All these hard tables of the past year have connected me to my frightening illness in a palpable way. They have been involved in its discovery and its treatment. The tables have followed me through the course of this nightmare, always present and uncomfortable. I deeply look forward to not lying on cold, uncomfortable tables in the future. Like so much about this experience, I hope that the feel of hard tables below my body will become just a memory, fading quickly into the stuff of dreams.

Miracles

 TRAVELING EAST ALONG INTERSTATE 10 about fifty miles
from Los Angeles, I spy it sitting like a mausoleum, dominating the surrounding structures and hillsides of the San
Bernardino Valley: Loma Linda University Medical Center. This flagship of the Seventh-Day Adventist hospital system was seemingly built
to satisfy a medical and spiritual vision of greatness. The off-cream
whiteness of its facades glows in the afternoon sun, setting it apart
from the drab greens and red-tiled roofs of surrounding homes. Two
gigantic circular wings flare out from its center, each eight stories high. It
is visible from more than ten miles away—quite a feat in the usually
hazy atmosphere of this Southern California megatropolis.

I ponder its image as I try to keep my rental car moving the requisite eighty miles per hour. The hospital complex rises like a spiritual
beacon on the landscape, and I steer toward it hoping for a taste of its
promised miracles.

In my days before this cancer, in my days of wellness, I would
often (perhaps more than normal) ruminate on what I would do when
faced with an uncompromising illness. Part of this came from being a
physician and seeing the full extent of the pathology that afflicts our
human species. I saw the rare, the tragic, the incomprehensible injustices

to innocents who suddenly developed maladies that would change everything forever. I saw the efforts they and their families invested in high-cost, high-tech medical procedures where the hint of cure was subtly offered yet rarely delivered. And as the long-term chair of our hospital's bioethics committee, I oversaw the process of families coping with the inevitable decision of when to stop the hoping and begin the grieving. Concepts like "quality of life" became benchmarks for not only bioethical considerations on behalf of others but my own mortality issues as well—whenever that time was to arrive in the dim future.

Well, the future has been here for the past year. I have a malignant and metastatic cancer. I have undergone countless CT scans and MRIs and arteriograms and blood studies. I have had two major surgeries that left me disabled and disfigured. I have undergone five weeks of conventional radiation therapy that so fried my neck, mouth, and throat that they literally bubbled down to germinal layers.

And now I am rushing on the California freeway toward this glowing monolith in the desert looking for a miracle of high-tech proportions. Here, three stories below the ground, encased in fifteen feet of lead and concrete, is the only regularly operated linear accelerator in the United States where elemental protons, the magic bullets of cancer treatment, are sent pulsating at the speed of light into deep, unapproachable tissues of the body. Looking for a cure, looking for a miracle.

I always thought that when faced with a critical scenario such as this, I would be logical and brave and insightful. I'd balance the probability of success with the downside of treatment courses. I'd be appropriately pensive given the diagnosis, and admirable in my resolve not to run scared. There would be a peaceful, cosmic rightness in my resignation, like accepting the cycles of seasons and the ever-changing expanse of clouds in Western skies.

Why, then, am I here? I'm here because of hopefulness. And a newfound belief in miracles.

I come from a history of miracles, although I lost the magic of anticipation decades ago. In my rigorous Roman Catholic upbringing, miracles—and praying for them—were hallmarks of my life. The saints, certified as such by their ability to foster miracles, were the beacons of our holy days, the names we took at confirmation, and the heavenly examples of how to live a pious life on earth. We prayed to St. Anthony for miracles in finding lost objects, St. Jude for lost causes, and St. Christopher for safe trips on long vacations in the family car.

But then I fell from grace, questioned the teachings of the church, and broke away completely—rejecting its tenets as elitist, sexist, and productive of unnecessary, unwarranted guilt. The day I purposefully missed my first Sunday Mass in twenty years, the promise of miracles as a possibility in life disappeared, along with my fearful commitment to the church's teachings.

My spiritual void was filled by the here-and-now dogma of existentialism. God was dead, and immediate reality reigned supreme. The universe, as I now saw it, was based on an organized chaos of molecular interactions, not on some grand design and spiritual icon sitting in a cloudy heaven. Both tragedies and sudden salvations from misery occurred randomly, not because of answers to prayers. Miracles were the stuff of life for those who needed crutches.

As years passed, my experiences softened that somewhat boring and nasty approach to making sense out of life's mysteries. The recreational use of mind-altering drugs in the '60s played a part. At that point the concept of a "separate reality" became a good friend. The universe became more wonderfully complex than the collision of oppositely charged molecules.

I subsequently spent a decade living and working with Native Americans in isolated reservation settings, where traditional ways were still practiced and one could feel how the earth, sky, rocks, and all living things were inexorably tied together in cycles of change. Spirituality returned to my life—not in the form of bearded biblical characters, but in the concept of a living energy that connected and nurtured all things.

And then came the reoccurrence of my cancer after twenty-six years. There is nothing like being faced with a potentially terminal illness to stimulate serious reflection on spirituality and miracles. The turnabout had little to do with grasping at straws during the final moments, requesting forgiveness for having fallen from the church's graces, or copping a plea for reinstatement before judgment time is at hand. I still have not returned to the Roman Catholic Church; when I pray, it is to the sky and my sense of Great Spirit instead of an Anglo-Saxon god image.

But facing this critical illness has produced long hours of wonderment on what life's about. Matters are still a bit muddy, as they tend to be with cosmic thoughts, yet the general essence of how a universal spirit connects with me during my brief time in this reality has become more comprehensible. And with it, the possibility of miracles has resurfaced.

Thinking back on this nightmarish year, I recall three moments in which I experienced terror at what I was facing. Certainly, for many more moments I've been emotionally down and pensive and pessimistic; but during three times of terror I felt scared to the core and looked for spiritual answers to help me escape from that frightening place.

The first was when the tumor recurrence was discovered. I knew something crazy was going on, with months of increasing pain, dizziness, and a rapidly enlarging lymph node in my neck. I asked a radiologist friend for a quick MRI on me one evening after a shift in the emergency room. The MRI was done hastily, unofficially, and his reading of the computer images came immediately, without leaving time for reflection or the digital augmenting that can provide so much more information. What he saw was simply old scar tissue from previous surgeries, whereupon I went home relieved.

The frightening moment came the next day when, having returned from running errands, I found a message on my answering machine to call my radiologist friend right away. Even before I dialed his number, fear penetrated my body and gripped my chest. He was apologetic, yet straight to the point. He had read the initial MRI too quickly—on further viewing, there was indeed a very troublesome, very large mass at my skull base that protruded into an opening in my skull and was putting critical pressure on my brain stem and spinal cord. Could I come back right away for another MRI? I knew at that second that this experience would overwhelm my days and nights for months if not years to come.

The next moment of numbing fear came four weeks later, on the day before I entered our hospital for neurosurgery. I was visiting the neurosurgeon who would be delicately fooling around with my brain the next morning. Up to that point, the prognosis most often given was that this malignancy would be manageable. But late that afternoon, with just the two of us in his office, he looked at me with his best professional detachment and said matter-of-factly that all he hoped to achieve the next day was removal of the small portion of tumor that was pressing on the brain stem. The rest of the sizable mass would be left alone, growing in its malignant potential, for he couldn't safely do any more than the intracranial work during one surgery. The complete removal, if such a feat were possible, would have to be staged in one or two additional operations.

I sat in silence, numb again with a primal feeling of helplessness that neither words nor comforting could dispel. The surgery the next day would not be the end of this nightmare, but rather the start of a series of hospitalizations, surgeries, and periods of convalescence. I do not remember a moment of the fifteen-mile journey back to my home that evening, so locked was my mind on other issues.

The third time of terror gripped me not long ago, as I was about to enter the radiation treatment phase. A full nine months had gone by since the initial neurosurgery, including five long months of recuperation from a thirteen-hour radical neck dissection at a major medical center in Dallas, for more removal of the malignant mass. I had spent the summer slowly healing from that second surgery, which left me compromised beyond all anticipation. But I was feeling better now, optimistic that radiation would be the final and complete treatment of this horrible condition. I had stopped feeling and acting like a patient.

As the radiation oncologist prepared to treat me, another MRI was conducted. After the study, I sat in the reading room while the X-ray sheets came out of the processor and were hung neatly on the banks of fluorescent view boxes. My old imaging studies from after the surgery in Dallas were also there for comparison.

The radiologist didn't have to point out what had occurred: the malignancy, now brightly lit by contrast material given intravenously during the study, was again massive on my skull base and working its way back into my intracranial area. It had almost doubled in size in just those five months since the "definitive surgery" in Dallas. This historically slow-growing tumor had through malignant changes become uncontrollably aggressive. Hence, the radiation treatment would not be a conservative zap, as was expected, to tie off loose ends and eradicate any microscopic cancer cells remaining after surgery, but a full-blown blast to arrest the growth of this persistent tumor before its effect on my brain was one of finality.

Again, a setback of fear that cut to the soul. Again, the necessity to reflect on my mortality and the spirit of the universe, which seemed something I was apt to experience sooner rather than later.

Now I find myself looking at the faces of other cancer patients at this California medical center so far from home. Many have come great distances, following the miracle path. Some are older men, obviously diagnosed with severe prostatic cancer, which is rumored to be treatable by proton therapy. Many are children, holding on to their parents' hands. Most are hairless from recent chemotherapy, wearing baseball caps to cover their wonderfully smooth heads. Some patients are in wheelchairs or using walkers, looking fragile and terminal. Still others, like me, appear relatively healthy despite the monster growing somewhere inside them. We mostly sit in silence, sharing wordlessly the secret of our individual journeys.

I notice a certain gleam in most of their eyes. There is a hopefulness, a *joie de vivre* that contradicts their condition. I hope they see a similar gleam in my eyes, I tell myself. The promise of miracles still lives in my heart, so it must be visible in my eyes.

My course is now lost in the future. I have undergone the treatments with vigor. The surgeries have been tolerated, and the two courses of radiation treatment completed. I'm told by the specialists that only time will tell. There is no point in having another imaging study right away, for it will show only the same-size tumor surrounded by swelling from the radiation treatment, which obscures whether or not its growth has been arrested. In three to four months another MRI will be helpful, although not conclusive. More imaging studies over six, nine, and twelve months will tell the tale. Until then, it's only a guess.

There is a possibility that in six months this tumor will again have doubled in size, posing a grim outlook. Or it might be the same size, or smaller, or nearly gone. No one can say except those in charge of miracles.

So my immediate choices are two: to either live with the frightening pessimism that all treatments have been for naught and my days are numbered, or accept that life, if only for the next few months, will go on punctuated by miracles at every moment.

Maybe taking the second course—no matter how difficult this may be—will help actualize the magic in the time that is left for me. Perhaps in the warm spirit of the cosmos, I will then find the peace I thought I'd be capable of before terror colored the reality of my days. I hope I have the courage to achieve such harmony, for that will be the most powerful proof that miracles do indeed exist.

Another
Recurrence

 IT'S COME BACK AGAIN. Just a few weeks since my surgery on that unexpected mass in the frontal lobe of my brain, another fast-growing tumor has appeared. The malignancy has returned.

I missed sensing this one. I've become fairly well versed in following the progress of this disease, finding new lumps or symptoms before they've been confirmed by an MRI. I've also hid my discoveries for weeks before reality forced me to get the imaging study, to seek follow-up.

But this tumor came as a big surprise. As someone who for the better part of twenty years has felt the contours of his neck, looking for telltale signs of new growth, how could I have missed it?

It was right there, in the front part of my neck, just above the larynx. A sizable, freely mobile, troublesome mass—it could not be anything other than a new metastatic lesion. And yet, I didn't consciously admit that it was there until the surgeon palpated it and said, without equivocation, "We have a problem here."

Why has this new mass forced a greater sense of finality than the six or seven other findings since December 1993? The subtle signs of this cancer tend to accumulate a certain intensity, to be sure, but what is it about this solitary mass in my neck that has struck such a deep chord of dread? Is it cumulative emotional fatigue from the relentlessness of this disease? Is it the short interval that has elapsed since the last big mass?

Events seem to be moving so quickly now. In the recent past, there was time for reflection—even optimism that the slow-growing malignancy could be arrested with a little surgery here, a little radiation there. Able to stay a stride ahead of each new lesion, I felt hopeful that despite the nastiness of this paraganglioma, I could revel in greater longevity, or at least postponement of the final reckoning.

But each time a new lesion developed in some far-removed location, without warning signs or symptoms, the inevitability of this illness hit me full-faced, arousing anger. Optimism and hope are growing dim. The time for acknowledgment, acceptance, and increased serenity is upon me.

Like everyone else, I don't want to die. Not knowing what the passage will bring, contemplating its uncertainty is a frightening experience. Often during my meditations and quiet reflections, I feel a peacefulness about the change between this existence and another. It feels much like a passage of joy, freedom from the struggles.

But such freedom is not certain. If it were, the peacefulness would remain. What lingers is fear that it may all be for nothing, that the fifty-some years of this existence will be forgotten in a flash. Those who have known me will undoubtedly spend a brief time in reflection and remembrance, and then move on with their lives, having no substantive thoughts of me in passing.

Why do I need a legacy of remembrance? Considering the long evolution of humankind, and still longer history of cosmic change, my brief time in this place doesn't deserve even a moment of reflection. I've been like countless other beings of the universe: we're here and then we're gone, with not a footprint left in the sand to show we ever existed.

Even so, I am hoping I have touched people in a way they will occasionally remember. I have tried to be available to listen, to empathize, to let others share fears, pains, joys, celebrations. I have attempted to spread healing rather than pain. I have endeavored to look at the greater purpose of the human condition, rather than groveling in its meanness. I have chosen to honor the laughter in my childhood, as opposed to the screams of pain and abuse.

But who will remember me for such things? Despite the momentary grieving of a few, will there be any legacy?

I am embarrassed by these ramblings of self-importance. I've always maintained great admiration for people of quiet strength who have rejected any sense of specialness in their lives. Those who protested against self-absorption had a lasting message for others. They were the first to say, "When I go, there need not be tears or sadness. Rather, the order of business is to move on, reflect on your own possibilities, and not dabble in memories."

So why, if these individuals have been so admirable to me, should I not remember their example at this time of potential finality? Why do I need such lasting importance now?

Just another mystery—strands of fear about facing personal mortality, with absolutely no control over the weaving.

Letter to
Chamisa

IN THE LATE 1970S I had a brief yet warm relationship with a Navajo nurse living in the Santa Fe area. A beautiful baby girl unexpectedly resulted from this liaison. I was not aware of her existence until a few weeks before she was born, then mother and daughter disappeared from my life.

For fifteen years I had no word of the child's situation, except indirect information that she was healthy, loved, and part of a solid family. Although I thought of her often, I did not seek her out, in keeping with her mother's request.

Then one evening in fall of 1994, I received a phone call at home. At the other end of the line, a soft, almost frightened voice introduced herself as my daughter Chamisa, long absent from my life. Within weeks we were meeting frequently and sharing time together with our mutual families. Now twenty years old, Chamisa is a college student embarking on a successful career as a fashion model. She and my son Adam have reveled in the discovery of a sibling they never knew existed. She has been a great source of strength for me during these years of health challenges. The following letter, written just before her seventeenth birthday, celebrates our newly found deep connection.

November 1996

Dear Chamisa:

I'm so glad you called to remind me of your approaching birthday. I remember the date well, but not well enough to plan ahead. I hope this note and card find you before the big day.

There are two special events, occurring during the weeks before I went into my most recent surgery, that I want to share with you. To share not so much for me, but for your understanding of things that are part of your history and place in time.

About two weeks ago I heard from a friend, Karen Waconda, a strong Isleta-Laguna Pueblo woman I work with in state government. She related that she had suddenly heard from an old friend named Bruce Gomez of Taos Pueblo. Bruce is a young spiritual leader in Taos who has worked most of his life with people of the northern pueblos. He is also well-known for his long-distance cross-country team, and for his expertise in the deep cultural connections between running and Indian spirituality. Bruce told Karen he was running alone the other day through the high mountains of Taos Pueblo, when he received a "message" of sorts about me, and that she was somehow associated with those thoughts. Bruce and I had met and worked together on pueblo youth issues about fifteen years ago, but had rarely seen each other since then. Soon after he finished running, he called Karen because of this feeling he had gotten about me. What does she know of me? he asked. He did not seem aware that Karen and I had been working together for the past two years. Karen told him of my health challenges and the most recent recurrence of the disease. Bruce asked her to bring me and him together, for the next weekend he and his father were leading a rarely held all-night ceremony of the Native American Church up in Taos, and he wanted to have the opportunity to pray for my situation at their important gathering.

I have no idea how much you know about the Native American Church, but it is a strong influence among many tribes around the country, with its combination of ancient Indian spirituality and common traditional medicine practices. Practitioners in the church run the spectrum from

*respected elders to young Indians trying to preserve the knowledge of tra-
ditional ways.*

*I didn't realize it initially, but Bruce's great-grandfather had
brought the Native American Church to Taos in the early 1900s from
tribes in the Dakotas; and from there its teachings had spread throughout
the Southwest to the Navajo and many other tribes in this area. Its spiritual
essence is a combination of old and new rituals. Meetings, or ceremonies,
take place only a few times a year, and consist of long sessions in sacred
tepees, beginning at dusk and lasting until dawn. There are extended
hours of prayers and ancient chants, consuming the sacred peyote, perhaps
being blessed with visions and getting in touch with the Great Spirit. At
dawn, with the sun rising over the mountains to the east, the ceremony
ends and the new day is welcomed with prayers and food.*

*I immediately called Bruce, since although we had not talked in
years, he obviously had received some sense of my situation through those
pathways of communication that defy explanation. He felt the weight of
my present problems, he said, and wanted to offer whatever prayers might
be helpful. He then invited me to join him at the close of the all-night ceremony in Taos.*

*At dawn that next Sunday, I awoke long before first light and traveled
alone to Taos. The home of Bruce's father was way back into pueblo land,
but I was eventually able to find it, and also locate the hundred-year-old
tepee of his grandmother, nestled among the cottonwood trees near the river.*

*Bruce and his father welcomed me into their sacred place as the
night-long ceremony was ending. The interior of the massive tepee was
dark, warm, and smelling sweetly of piñon wood and sage. A few members
of the meeting were reclining along the periphery of the tepee, watching but
not challenging my presence in that space. I was asked to walk around the
fire they had been keeping all night, and to touch the wet earth around
the coals that had been the source of their prayers those many hours. Bruce
and his father spent time with me that morning, saying prayers in their
language, spreading sacred cedar smoke on me, touching me with falcon
feathers that had been in their family for generations. I felt at home and
blessed in their presence. After the ceremony, I joined their families and*

children under the cottonwoods in a feast of many foods. Bruce's mother, I learned that morning, is a Navajo who has been in Taos almost thirty years. She gave me a big hug. Bruce and I spoke little, knowing we had connected in a way important to us both.

The next weekend, a ceremony took place at my house. Again, my friend Karen Waconda helped broker it, through a Native American psychiatrist from Albuquerque named Irv Lewis, who despite his impressive credentials in Western medicine, is a traditional Navajo healing man. He helped put together a ceremony run by a wonderful woman named Elsie Kahn. Elsie is a middle-aged Navajo healer who was for many years an ordinary secretary with the tribe, just going through the motions like so many of us. She was faced with lots of illness in her life and tragedy within her family. She said she was once taking fourteen different medications. Then seven years ago, she began to have a series of intense dreams and spiritual messages. After fighting them off for a long time, she went to a medicine person in Navajoland to ask some questions and was told she must go to the Dakotas for the answers. She quit work and traveled north, where she was greeted by people who told her she was expected. Eventually, they sent her back to her land, where she spent much time in the mountains and was visited by the eagle that gave her duties and powers.

This is not my story; it comes from her.

So she stopped working and began her journey as a healer. According to Irv Lewis, traditional Navajo people feel that she has great power.

Elsie traveled all the way from Window Rock, Arizona, to join me in our home on Saturday morning. She and her husband, Raymond (who had worked for Indian Health Service more than twenty-four years), and their young grandson, Kyle, arrived in a red, mud-coated pickup truck. Irv Lewis and Karen Waconda from Albuquerque joined us soon afterward. My wife Barbara and her mother, Irene, were there as well. Early in the morning, I had built a large fire to warm the place and prepare coals for the ceremony.

Elsie Kahn is a humble and powerful woman. She gathered the few of us in a circle on the floor and placed coals from the fire on a bed of earth from outside. She started the ceremony by covering the coals with dry cedar, which ignited into a plume of sweet-smelling smoke that filled the room. She talked about herself, and how she came to this place. Then I spoke of my prayers and wishes for this ceremony. Following that, everyone else had a chance to speak briefly about why they came.

Between herself and the glowing coals on the floor, Elsie opened a white linen cloth that held a few crystals, other stones, and an eagle feather. She prayed in the Navajo language for some time, spreading cedar and sage on the coals every so often. Raymond followed with a long prayer of healing. Elsie then spoke of my illness, which she seemed to know about in detail without any information beforehand. She looked into the coals and talked about my past, the upcoming surgery, and what my future might hold. She began to shake and softly moan with the intensity of things she was feeling. She spoke in comforting yet realistic terms. This was not so much a healing ceremony of the body as one that blessed the spirit and allowed me to face whatever might be there for me in the future.

With her eagle feather, she then spread cedar smoke over me and touched my neck and back and arms with a healing stroke, all the time intoning that she sensed a long sickness was going to continue for me. In our own way we all prayed together.

As time passed in silence, Elsie asked me to look into the glowing coals and tell her what I saw. It was as clear to me as watching a movie on TV. In the coals that morning, I clearly saw my face—my face with a large smile on it. That was the message she got as well. No matter what happened with this thing, smiles and laughter were going to be part of it.

Soon afterward, she closed the ceremony. I was then asked to spread the coals and earth around the entire periphery of my house. So I walked alone outside that cool morning and sent the ashes and brown earth back from where they came. I smiled the whole way.

Soon afterward, we had a big meal of posole and green chile stew and tortillas. I gave various people gifts and blankets to thank them for coming and taking part in the ceremony. We laughed a lot about kids and other things. In the early afternoon, Elsie and Raymond and their grandson moved on to Cochiti Pueblo, after which I found myself smiling constantly for quite a while.

This is again a crazy time, like those days we spent a few years ago when I first saw you. When I say that my spirit feels good, it is a true feeling, even though so much uncertainty lies in the future. You and I and our families have come together at a late stage in my life, and a rapidly changing one in yours. Still, it is better that we came together now instead of never having had the chance to come together at all.

Happy birthday. I look forward to seeing you at Christmastime. Keep in touch with your brother Adam, please. He, like I, feels a great importance in you.

Love,

Tim

Last Surgery

AFTER MY FIFTH MAJOR SURGERY, I looked at myself in the mirror and wondered how I got to this place. It seemed that only an instant ago I was vibrant and alive with solid health. Then I began to get whittled down. An initial surgery to remove the tumor on my brain stem. An unexpected lapse from postoperative meningitis. Preparation for further surgery in Dallas, with frequent trips to that obnoxious city—study after study, airplane after airplane. Finally, successful attempts to shut off blood supply to the skull-based tumor and a major fifteen-hour operation by a team of famous surgeons. Not one surgeon—no one's capable of doing it alone—but a team of them. A full-press effort by the best that Texas had to offer. Weeks in the hospital feeling beaten and abused, and then home for a long convalescence.

After the physical healing, it was time to enter the world of radiation. More studies, CAT scans, measurements for precise exposure to the mass. Be sure we don't miss a millimeter of calculation or we'll fry the brain stem like a fresh egg on a skillet. Weeks and weeks of radiation, alone in that isolated, sterile room with the electric whine of machinery and ticking of internal clocks. It's an unseen world—not like real surgery, where the blood and tumors and crisp, staccato sounds of the surgeon's orders are palpable, but rather invisible, mysterious, electro-magnetic, unimaginable. The skin tells the hidden story. The skin on the neck begins to flake, then dissolve into primal cells and screaming pestilence. I leave each radiation session with a dream that the tumor is feeling a similar pain.

Then long, isolated trips to the white temple in the desert of California—Loma Linda Medical Center. A promise of mortality with the highest of high tech. A proton accelerator, the only one regularly operating in the nation, which sends magic bullets deep inside tissues to zap the last of renegade cells. Long days and nights spent alone in cold motels in the valley. Dutifully getting up each day to lie on the hard, sterile table in the bowel of the accelerator. Sessions of only ten minutes, then days of waiting for the next encounter, all the while sur-rounded by plaques and art and testimonies to the money it took to produce this edifice of modern medicine.

So the treatment has come to an official end. It's wait-and-see time—difficult at best, impossible in some moments. Waiting for another MRI and waiting for Godot.

At about the time of Christian high religion—Good Friday, Easter, and all—a follow-up MRI is done, with results to follow a few days later. Barbara and I take a long walk to the ancient shrine in Chimayo, as if this pilgrimage celebrating Christian principles has any relevance to where I find myself. But walk I do, pretending this brand of prayer is important.

The results of the MRI look surprisingly good. Little growth of the primary tumor; no new growth seen. An unexpected reprieve. Carry on, go forth, do not pass this way again.

I try that route. I really try that optimistic route. I enter into work, into a resurgence of my profession, an ignorance of the past. Although the physical manifestations remain, the spirit stays strong. My illness becomes past history as I move along.

Then the inevitable recurrence takes place. An enlarged cancerous node is discovered under my left jaw, which I consciously ignore for months except in moments of dreams and solitude. It—and what it represents—will not go away. I finally accede to tests and further study. It is indeed a new lesion, an offspring of the one that came before.

More consultations, more preparation, more surgery. This time the intervention is quick and focused. One day of outpatient surgery—in and out. Under the gas, remove the gland and nodes, sew up the incision, and get him home by dinnertime.

Despite the implications, it all feels surprisingly benign. I heal at home for a week, then return to the fray as if nothing unusual has happened.

For months on end I continue the charade of work and future, though the nagging image of mortality lingers in my brain. Nowhere is truly safe. No long-range plans are possible. Dreams of seeing children grow up and plans accomplished are simply that—dream material.

Six months after the second recurrence, I endure a routine MRI to please the oncologist, who lives on data and evidence. Surprisingly, to everyone except myself, the MRI shows a new and troublesome lesion far removed from the primary one, invading the frontal lobe of my brain.

It is now the time of decision. If I succumb to fatigue from it all, I'll opt to do nothing and let the new tumor grow until it sends my brain stem screaming into the foramen magnum as I die from paralysis, asphyxiation, and pain. If I agree to the surgery, it is another painful round of hospitalization, physical insult, convalescence, and the self-consciousness that comes from being the dependent patient. What mutually unacceptable alternatives these seem to be!

It is one thing to accept the natural course of a progressive disease and reach the reasonable conclusion that enough is enough. But pressure from others—family and heath providers—becomes a loud voice for action, no matter how fruitless it may seem. It's only an isolated node in the frontal lobe, I'm reminded. There is no sign of further extension. Let's just pop it out and see what happens. What is there to lose?

Then there is the voice of my own spirit to live, which grows stronger with each new challenge, each new appearance of a tumor mass. I sometimes overlook how afraid I am to die. At least if there is a chance, I tell myself, any chance at all.

So the surgery date is set. Another relatively quick admission and discharge from the hospital—including two days or so in-hospital as my friend the neurosurgeon saws out a circular entranceway into the frontal bone above my eyebrow and removes the handball-size mass. People come to visit at my hospital bed, expressing the familiar hollow greeting: "My, don't you look wonderful. I can't believe you just had brain surgery."

I make jokes and entertain them with optimism, although most is generated by the high-dose mind-altering steroids dripping from my IV rather than any inherent feelings of confidence.

Again, a brief time at home recuperating, then back to work with the state Department of Health and the University Medical School. I wear a baseball cap almost constantly as I return to those professional settings, trying to hide the ear-to-ear semicircular incision and the irregular patches of shaven hair left by the surgery. People, as always, are supportive, but we all know that these past four years have marked me as someone with a progressive, ubiquitous illness that is forever my companion.

Three months later, at a routine checkup, yet another metastatic mass is discovered in the front of my neck, near the vocal cords. It wasn't detectable on the MRIs a few months before, or by the surgeon's trained hands as they palpated critical areas. This time there are no deliberations. Let's just cut this baby out right away, I declare, and not ask any big bioethical questions. It's a fight, and I'm in it to the end.

Another quick day-surgery to remove the malignant node, and home in time to watch *Sport Center*. The incision is barely two inches long and heals quickly, leaving few signs that I've had more surgery.

But then one morning I look at myself in the mirror as I prepare to head off to work. It's not that quick glance at the reflection we are accustomed to taking nearly every morning of our lives; rather, it becomes a long, intense, almost hallucinogenic stare at my own face. I gaze at the remnants of scars on my forehead and neck, some resembling architectural plans for superhighway intersections, with crossing patterns and double loops. I look at the left side of my neck, now barely a third of its former size, disfigured by a grotesque crater from below my ear to my collarbone. Forcing a smile, I look at the abnormal curve of my lower lip, distorted from the frequent facial nerve damage. But most of all, I look at my eyes—beyond the cornea and colored iris, into the link between the wondrous orbs and the core of the soul. Deep down there, I see unmistakable sadness and resignation. I see the future.

"That will be my last surgery," I hear myself saying. I may agree to a touch of radiation treatment to stave off the progression to the other side of my neck, if it seems at all hopeful. But I am done with surgery. After all, I have long viewed this journey with cancer as a mutual contention between conflicting-yet-natural processes, not as a "war" that should be "waged" to the end.

I want to live. My malignancy wants to live. We both use what's available to us to achieve those ends, much like the ying and yang of Eastern cosmologies. Contrasting yet ever blending black and white, peace and war, good and evil, insight and confusion. At one and the same time, the most evil of things can also be a blessing of new knowledge and growth. On and on the cycles will continue, always changing.

Definitely, I will have no more surgery for this thing. No more.

Vision Quest

It is called by many names. To the Sioux it is *hanblecheya*, the "crying for a vision" time. Aborigines from Australia call it walkabout. Each culture has its own version of the ritual, and although every one of them is unique, they share a core similarity.

The vision quest. A critical time when a young person moves from one path to another. A necessary ordeal of isolation and discovery; a singular path one must take to reach a new level of understanding and spirituality. It is a time of danger, perhaps even death, as the young one goes off alone into wild places and faces severe sacrifices so that the visions may come. Those visions lead the way to future directions and important decisions.

During the isolation and physical hardships of a vision quest, the hope is that the person will be visited by a spiritual messenger, usually in the form of an animal, bird, or physical event, that will serve as a guide in future days. Occasionally, the spirit messenger will not appear, and instead, an unquestionable understanding will arise of the way things are. And sometimes nothing will evolve from the quest except pain, fear, and more confusion. Whatever the details may be, no one returns from a vision quest without having undergone some fundamental change.

I thought often of the vision quest as I prepared for a marathon-like bicycle trek across New Mexico.

The young Republican governor of New Mexico, a political novice, came out of nowhere to win the statehouse in a reaction to Democrats' blunders over a number of years. A self-made millionaire in his early forties, he was known as a physical fanatic who exercised vigorously before dawn seven days a week and competed in marathons and iron-man contests. Every year after his election, he would lead a week-long bicycle journey across the large state to heighten public awareness of trash on the roadsides. Called "Trek for Trash," the 1997 ride was a good PR opportunity and a chance for him to officially practice his biking skills for an upcoming ironman competition in Hawaii. Just as important, it got him away from constant battles with Democratic legislative leaders in Santa Fe, to mingle with the rural folks who had elected him to office. It was a relatively no-lose situation for the young governor.

Through administrative channels, the directive came down from the governor's office to the state Department of Health that some on-site emergency response should be provided—God forbid that the governor or members of his entourage should stub their toes while on the five-day journey. The directive trickled down to the Emergency Medical Services Bureau, where I was the state medical director, to supply that coverage. It was an easy task: get a seasoned paramedic from the bureau, outfit a van with critical emergency equipment, set up communication linkages with local EMS transport services and hospitals along the route, and simply have the van follow the pack of bicyclists on their long journey.

As medical director, I was responsible for determining what equipment and supplies should be on board, establishing connections with local hospitals, and making myself available by radio or phone to provide direct "medical control" to the paramedic should a major emergency occur. But then something happened.

One evening as I sat on my front porch watching the late-summer clouds produce a magical display of changing shapes and colors against the setting sun, an intense thought visited me: Why not go on the ride myself—not as a passenger in the trailing emergency van moving at ten miles an hour behind the bicyclists, but as a rider? Intense thoughts often came as I watched clouds move across endless skies, but this one seemed more foolish than most. Nevertheless, the more I contemplated the activity of the clouds, the more this idea took on the dimensions of a distinct possibility.

I had a fairly functional, moderately expensive road bike. Although hardly one of the high-tech, space-age bicycles of competitive racers, it had served me well on occasional long rides around northern New Mexico. I wasn't by any means an accomplished bicyclist—the longest trek I had ever undertaken was sixty miles—but I frequently took ten- to twenty-mile recreational jaunts when time and weather allowed.

The proposed journey, however, was nothing like an easy weekend ride a few miles from home. This was to be a physically challenging, incredibly intense five-day journey of 533 miles from the northwest to southeast borders of the fifth largest state in the nation. Although there would be occasional rest stops to replenish fluids and food, the daily treks would start before dawn and end in early evening with scheduled distances of 100 to 120 miles a day. The route would traverse high mountain passes of more than 7,000 feet, cross the Continental Divide, and pass through long stretches of open, harsh desert.

What was I possibly thinking about?

I was thinking about the vision quest. I desperately needed the challenge that this trip represented. For four years I had been contending with the physical and emotional nightmares sparked by a rare malignancy. There had been five major surgeries, four long radiation treatments, and countless months of slow rehabilitation. For a while, the cancer appeared to have been effectively treated; then over the previous eight months, three unexpected tumors had emerged far from the original site. My most recent surgery had taken place only six weeks earlier, when a malignant node was removed from under my jaw. I was now facing the certainty of progressive disease and a resultant uncertainty about the future. I was scheduled for an eight-week last-ditch course of radiation to my neck—a treatment I was ambivalent about. My active life as a respected emergency physician had come to an abrupt halt, and there was even doubt that I would be able to continue my administrative position with state government or my faculty teaching duties at the medical school in Albuquerque. Short, short horizons and lack of expectations were themes I lived with every day.

The answer was obvious as I watched my friends the clouds. Take the bike trip. What could it do—kill me? Perhaps something important would come to me during the quest, especially while I searched for spiritual answers to the uncertainties that plagued me.

DAY ONE—MONDAY

The journey began in Gallup, at the far west side of the state. Gallup is a classic Indian reservation "border town" I had come to know well over the previous twenty years. Although a longtime railroad, commercial, and mining center, Gallup's real raison d'être, like that of so many towns on the edge of Indian land, was to provide both sustenance and misery to its Native American neighbors—in this case, the Navajo and Hopi to the northwest and the Zuni to the south. The seedy main street of town displays a strip of pawnshops interspersed with down-and-out bars and tragically inebriated Indians passed out in the alleys and open parks. What a bizarre jumping-off place, I reflected wryly as we drove the streets of Gallup toward the trek's starting point.

I had arrived the previous evening with my friend Fred, a paramedic from our bureau. We had attended the requisite ceremonial dinner for the governor, along with all local and Indian officials of a variety of political persuasions. In a sparsely populated state like New Mexico, any chance to be seen with and catch the ear of the governor is typically embraced.

I had slept fitfully in anticipation of the early-morning start. All night long, loud trains rolled by my motel room on their journey from Los Angeles to Chicago and beyond. As I listened to the click-clack of wheels on tracks and the drone of the big diesel engines, I recalled that people were often moving someplace else, seeking something else—the restless American saga.

The morning began before dawn. Even though mid-September days grow quite warm in these southern deserts, at 5:30 A.M. and at 6,500 feet above sea level, a numbing coldness pierced the thin synthetic material of my biking shorts and top. A large crowd was gathered at the city park to officially send off the governor and his group. High school cheerleaders in short skirts tried to stay warm by going through their orchestrated routines. The local radio station had a remote setup, with the morning DJ interviewing the governor and other dignitaries. Warm coffee and obscene numbers of cream doughnuts were passed among the crowd. I shivered alongside the EMS van as we made logistical connections with the three state police officers assigned to accompany the governor for the next five days.

After a few official words and photo ops for the local press, our cadre of bicyclists—perhaps only fifteen in number—majestically pedaled off through an arching banner of balloons and colored paper as the local high school marching band played on. I felt more like a participant in a small-town parade than a solitary soul embarking on a spiritual quest to find answers to the universe's great mysteries.

This comical beginning to my journey became even more surreal moments later. As we rode through the streets of Gallup, about a quarter-mile from the park my bike sped over a hidden pothole, causing my delicate rear tire to blow out. With more than 500 miles to go, I had lasted less than one lap around a high school track.

The pack of bikers was well out of sight by the time I pulled over to assess the damage. My spare tire tubes were in the van with Fred, who by then was miles ahead. I walked with my disabled bike through the early-morning deserted streets of Gallup, feeling utterly foolish. Luckily, I was overtaken by a nice elderly man driving one of the support vehicles for the two senior citizens on the trip, and he helped me throw my now-useless bike in the back of his van. Then we drove out of town to catch up with the pack at the first designated rest stop.

As the van moved toward Zuni Pueblo, I sat in it silently,

embarrassed and frustrated by this less-than-heroic beginning. Any thoughts of a grand spiritual adventure seemed to have blown up as quickly as my rear tire.

We caught up with the pack about fifteen miles south of Gallup, where it had stopped for the first of countless unplanned sojourns to pick up trash along the road. Here was the governor in all his self-centered fineness, walking along the rough back roads of New Mexico with white vinyl trash bags in hand, picking up a sordid collection of beer cans, old bottles, rain-soaked pieces of cardboard, and items that defied description. The governor prided himself on the tons of trash that would be gathered during the five-day journey, and had set a personal goal of collecting more on this trip than on the one the year before. I wondered if he worked as hard on the affairs of state as on this compulsive cleanup that would be his business for the next few days.

Fred and his van were nowhere to be found. So I scrounged among the other riders for anyone who had a spare tire to lend, and was finally able to find an agreeable fit. In a few minutes I was back on the road again, although now far behind the core pack of riders, who were in much better shape and had more sophisticated bikes. But at least I was riding. The day was quickly warming, and I felt sweat drip from beneath my biking helmet.

Our first official stop was on the border of Zuni Pueblo land, where members of the tribe had set up a station of traditional foods, fresh water, and fruit. Zuni Pueblo, consistently inhabited for almost a millennium, is called Sunyi'tsi in its people's native language.

Zuni's first nonnative visitor was a black slave named Estevanico, a guide for an expedition led by the Spanish missionary-explorer Fray Marcos de Niza in 1539. Ranging ahead of the main party in his role as scout, Estevanico entered the pueblo with an escort of Indians from other tribes. But he abused the Zunis' hospitality, taking liberties with their women and their stores of turquoise; and they subsequently killed him. Word of the murder frightened Fray Marcos, who did not follow his guide into the pueblo, but only glimpsed it from afar—and then went back with the mistaken report that he had discovered

Cíbola, the fabled Seven Cities of Gold. To most Zuni members, the history of their proud and peaceful people has gone downhill since that first, unwelcomed contact with a strange foreigner.

Our biking entourage devoured the wonderful red and green chile stews, freshly baked traditional bread, and large bowls of pudding and Jell-O. As people mingled about, I noticed a distinguished Indian man standing alone by a pickup truck. I immediately recognized him as the governor of Zuni Pueblo, an appointment designated anew each year by the spiritual hierarchy of the tribe. Resting in one hand, as if part of him, was the Lincoln cane.

The Lincoln cane is a 134-year-old relic presented to the tribal leader of each pueblo by President Lincoln in 1863, as a sign of respect and to solidify the treaties under negotiation. Since then, the same cane has been passed down from leader to leader, with the under-standing that it will be brought out only on very special occasions. I stared at the almost jet-black, smoothly finished mahogany wood and glowing engraved gold cap nestled in the pueblo governor's hand.

Approaching him, I briefly paid my respects and thanked his people for their gifts of food and water. He gave me a warm smile. What does he make of this strange display before him? I wondered. These grown men in tight Lycra shorts, brightly colored shirts, and funny little shoes talking among themselves at a dusty rest stop.

After the nourishment, our pack of riders headed directly south on the narrow rural highway to our next official rest stop in Fence Lake, about thirty-seven miles away. Soon the relatively flat foothills gave way to increasingly higher red-earth plateaus and then the pine-covered Zuni Mountains. Although the highway would take occa-sional descents, most of the time we were biking uphill through mile-long stretches of constant rises, where the lowest bike gears were needed just to keep moving.

At that point, the accomplished riders were out of sight and well ahead of me. No matter how much I forced my legs to move quickly, I fell farther and farther behind. I remembered the lecture that the trip organizer had given us the evening before the start—that the chase vehicle would be required to pick up all those who fell more than ten miles behind the main pack of riders. Hence I found myself fighting not only the ever ascending road into these beautiful mountains but also the fear that I would be plucked up by a chase vehicle as someone who wasn't able to cut it. So I pedaled harder, and became more winded. The constant burn in my legs grew more intense. What I had embarked on was no longer the stuff of a mystic quest; it was purely and simply a trip of pain and frustration.

I pushed myself into rhythmic breathing and a silently repeated mantra, which I hoped would sustain me on these hills for the miles to come. Instead of looking toward the endless mountain passes ahead, I centered on my breathing, or the feel of cool wind on my face, or the sweet smells of fall-blooming chamisa bushes. This hypnotic state, as it turned out, had enough self-produced endorphins to dull the burning in my legs and chest.

Eventually, I rolled into Fence Lake, a small farming community settled by refugees from the Dust Bowl in the early 1930s. All the other riders had arrived long before, eaten a lunchtime snack, and begun to seat up for the next leg of the trip. I limped into the rest stop at the local fire station feeling exhausted, faint, and discouraged. Aware that I had overextended myself to keep up with the governor and his accomplished pack, I reluctantly decided to replenish my reserves before further challenging my body.

I threw my bike into the back of Fred's van and grabbed some fruit and water bottles from the tables in front of the firehouse. I silently downed three bottles of water and a variety of fruit while Fred drove slowly behind the riders. Gradually, the fluid and fruit returned strength to my constitution, whereupon my dizziness and shaking began to dissipate.

About ten miles down the road, the pack stopped for another requisite trash-picking venture. The day had grown warm and most riders had shed layers of clothing. They were now wearing only biking shorts and brightly colored racing shirts. I felt rejuvenated from my rest and nourishment, and decided to rejoin the bikers for the next leg of the journey. After collecting another thirty bags of trash, the group headed off for the final thirty miles of the first day, and evening rest in the village of Quemado.

The late afternoon ride through those dramatic mountains of western New Mexico was moving. The brightly colored aspen and other seasonal trees contrasted with the dark greens of pine and juniper. The highway was virtually devoid of autos, so long stretches of solitary and wonderfully quiet riding provided welcome relief from the morning's ordeal. The earth and sky shimmered with beauty.

The last five miles into Quemado were on a moderate decline from the mountains. I floated through this last stretch almost with the delusion of being on the Tour de France. The first day on this journey has certainly been challenging, I mused. There were moments when I nearly decided to quit, to accept that the body can be urged to do only so much before it rebels. But with the ease of this last leg, images of the beauty of isolated mountains and high plains stayed with me, erasing those memories of pain. I remember hearing the ravens and occasional hawks flying overhead, and spying a lone deer moving through the trees just on the edge of the road. I had received no visions, been visited by no messengers, and heard no answers to my queries of the universe. Still, it had been a day rich with experiences.

That evening the community of Quemado, named after the Spanish word for "burned," hosted us to a home-cooked meal in the high school gym. An impromptu volleyball game between the governor's staff and local teachers brought out most of the villagers. Youngsters stood in line to have the governor autograph their T-shirts. It was small-town entertainment at its best.

I walked back early to Quemado's ancient and only operational motel, where I downed large doses of ibuprofen to combat the deep aches before quickly falling asleep. A moment before consciousness left, I could hear loud conversations outside my door, as riders and support staff began partying late into the night. I didn't know these people and didn't feel connected with them. Except for Fred, I was alone on this journey—as it should be for the solitary quest I was on.

Day Two—Tuesday

Again I was up before the first light of day. Although Gallup had been chilly, the predawn temperature in this mountain community was downright intolerable. While gathering at the forest ranger station just east of the village, we huddled around propane camping stoves and downed cup after cup of hot coffee and rock-hard pop tarts. With my jaw nearly frozen, chewing the dull pastries was almost impossible.

Riders slowly began pedaling away from Quemado, heading directly east toward the Datil Mountain Range. Trying to avoid a repeat of the previous day's embarrassing last-place finish, I took off before the main pack, to establish whatever head start I could. As the morning sun cut across the eastern horizon and began its warming of the earth, I could sense the sweet smells of dawn in this high land. The riding felt smooth and easy, and soon I again found myself entering a meditative rhythm of breathing and silent chanting.

But not for long. My peaceful musings were interrupted by the first casualty of the journey. A biker ahead of me, a young man from Gallup who had joined us for this leg of the trip, had experienced a sudden "lock" of his knee, causing him to take an unexpected violent trajectory over his handlebars and crash to the rough roadside. I came upon him soon after the event, and immediately switched internal gears to be the emergency physician rather than the solitary seeker.

As I assessed his injuries and asked key questions about any hidden problems, two things became obvious. First, that except for a strained knee and a few brushes of road burns on his elbows, he was not seriously injured. And second, that he was a young man challenged with a developmental disability of some sort, so I found it necessary to communicate with him at an age level much lower than his body's years would suggest.

Fred soon arrived in the emergency van, followed closely by the young man's mother in a new pickup truck. I reassured her that he was going to be fine although his day's ride would be cut short. She quickly acknowledged his disability and his excitement at riding with the governor, which may have caused him to overexert himself. We splinted his leg and arranged for his mother to return him to Gallup, where he could be more thoroughly checked at the hospital. The ingrained emergency practitioner in me made the requisite roadside diagnosis: probable slipped medial meniscus, likely a chronic problem he'd had for years. But I also wondered if he had subconsciously understood the great physical difficulties he would face that day, and conveniently taken an acceptable exit by flying off the bike. Does he have more courage than I, who yesterday would have longed for an "easy out" upon feeling I could no longer continue? I asked myself.

The governor and his cadre soon pedaled up to our little emergency in the wilderness and, like most rubbernecking passersby, began asking too many questions and exhibiting a hint of concern that Fred and I didn't know what we were doing. Things are under control, Governor—please ride on. Everything is fine. We have been here before.

By the time the young man was heading back to Gallup with his mother, the main pack was miles ahead, so I opted to throw my bike in the van and ride on with Fred to the next stop. Unlike the previous day, when the van offered salvation to my failing body, this time it provided an unwanted diversion from my energizing early-morning pedal through the beautiful countryside.

We soon arrived at another roadside trash-gathering detail, which gave me a chance to rejoin the pack. As we took off, the air started to warm up, and the ride felt rejuvenating, with only minor inclines as we rose toward the Datil Mountains. At one point, my vision locked on a unusual, impressive summit just to the south of our route: Escondido Peak. Once an incredibly high volcanic mountain, Escondido Peak is still almost 10,000 feet in elevation after millions of years of erosion. The timelessness of both this little orb we call earth and the universe flew around in my head, again giving perspective to the minuscule journey I was undertaking.

Our next official rest stop was in the small mountain community of Pie Town—so named for a baker who settled there in the late 1800s and was famous for his pie-making skills, which were enjoyed by early travelers and road workers alike. His grandson reportedly still lives in the village, although it is not known if he likes to bake. Again, more home-cooked pancakes and bitter coffee at the fire station, with opportunities for the governor to press the flesh with his kind of folks.

Leaving Pie Town, we headed up a steep road to the village of Datil, about twenty-one miles to the east. We were approaching the Continental Divide, that mysterious, unseen vertical line that runs down the spine of the North American continent—from high up in the wilderness of Alaska to the mountains of Central America and then onward through South America—and marks the division between water flow to the Atlantic and Pacific Oceans. I remembered learning about the Continental Divide as a youngster in school, and thinking how magical it would be to straddle that imaginary line, delicately placing separate drops of water just to the east and west of it, then follow them down their separate drainage paths, one leading to the Rio Grande and Gulf of Mexico, the other to the mighty Colorado River and on to the Sea of Cortez in Mexico. Now that's a dividing line, I told myself.

My fond remembrances from school days were quickly squelched by the here-and-now reality that this leg of the journey was taking us upward over ever-sharper inclines. The long climb up hill after hill seemed endless, and again I fell well behind the group, except for a senior citizen just behind me. My legs burned as the pace slowed and each rotation of the pedals became more difficult than the one before. Memories of Monday's trials and frustrations rushed over me. Again I worked consciously on my breathing, and tried to center on the beauty of these mountains bred from ancient volcanoes.

Somehow the meditative discipline kept me moving forward into Datil, an old stagecoach stop settled in 1884 and named, like the tall mountains surrounding it, from the Spanish word for "date," because the seedpods of the broad-leaved yucca plant growing nearby resembled the dates that grew in the old country. Or perhaps the early settlers were frustrated because they couldn't find female companions on Friday nights.

The road out of Datil was luxuriously invigorating. Downhill we soared on long sweeps of curves. Bikes were set in the highest gears, allowing us to move along at great speeds with only minimal pedaling. Cool breezes evaporated any remaining sweat. There was no need to enter into a meditative trance on this stretch. I was flying, full of energy, feeling invulnerable.

This long, sloping descent took us into an intriguing, almost mystical place called the Plains of San Augustín. This broad basin, almost eighty miles across, lies between the Datil and San Mateo Mountains. Millions of years ago it held a fifty-mile-long lake, the residence of dinosaurs. Closer to modern times, a large meteorite crashed into the plain, leaving a wealth of rocks from the heavens.

Right in the middle of this vast flatland was an otherworldly sight, visible from fifty miles away as we came down from the Datil Range. At first, my mind had difficulty processing what my eyes were seeing, for after the overwhelming eons-old natural beauty of the previous 180 miles of biking, I was gazing directly into the future, at a startling, gigantic piece of space-age technology: the Very Large Array, or VLA, as it is known to the locals.

VLA is the internationally known National Radio Astronomy Observatory portrayed in backdrops of such movies as *Star Trek* and *Contact*. Spread out over hundreds of square miles are twenty-seven huge radio antennas, each exactly eighty-two feet in diameter and weighing 235 tons. These massive dishes are all brilliant white, with the central receiving core pointed toward the heavens. The antennas are strategically aligned on three thirteen-mile railroad tracks arranged in a Y shape, so that by moving the dishes either closer to or farther away from the center, the collective radio telescope can range from 2,000 feet to thirteen miles in diameter. If the array were one dish instead of many, it would need to be seventeen miles in diameter to achieve the same sensitivity to signals from afar.

VLA was built to look not at the visual universe, but rather at the invisible substance of celestial events—the electromagnetic waves coming from quasars or novas or new galaxies in the making, generated millions to billions of years ago and just now reaching the earth. In addition to its purely scientific mission to look at events in the far reaches of the universe, VLA is also "listening" quietly for more cosmic footprints, the unmistakable pattern of radio waves that could only have been generated by an intelligent, advanced civilization from the stars. In short, VLA is looking for the others out there.

Our biking group stopped for a scheduled rest along the road at the entrance to VLA, some five miles east of Datil on the open plain. Greeting us were a group of pleasant upper-echelon observatory staff members happy to answer questions about their work. One quiet, unassuming older gentleman, dressed in jeans and a simple workshirt, came up to me and introduced himself. He turned out to be the director of the entire operation, a distinguished PhD in the field of radioastronomy. I immediately felt comfortable with his almost boyish enthusiasm for his work. Here was a man whose life was spent dreaming of civilizations in worlds millions of light-years away when our earth was still a bubbling inferno of volcanic activity. The quest of these radio astronomers touched me with its inexplicable enormity. These scientists have talked to the stars. What have they heard? What was the message?

From our brief encounter with the realm of black holes, we pressed on across the Plains of San Augustín, and began the hard climb into the Magdalena Mountains. Again I tried to get out far ahead of the pack, but within a few miles the governor and his competitive racers blew by me as if I were pedaling backward. The governor called out a brief encouragement—"Great job! Keep on going!"—which would become the predominant dialogue between him and me over those days. As the ascent became steadily steeper, I was also passed by an overweight middle-aged man and a white-haired senior citizen. They all blew by me, leaving me near the end of the pack again. With that, my mantra changed to a down-to-earth "Get me outta here!"

The town of Magdalena is one of those mining settlements that boomed in the late 1800s and is now struggling to survive with little or no local economy. Once, it was the center of these parts, known for having more bars and brothels than churches. Some $9 million worth of silver and lead ore was shipped out of Magdalena during its twenty-two-year heyday. The Magdalena Mountains surrounding the town on three sides are rugged and treeless, revealing their volcanic birth and a richness of silver, lead, malachite, and barite. Their harsh beauty otherwise escaped me as I struggled up the last few switchbacks and painfully rolled into town.

Magdalena had another big turnout for the governor's arrival. Various political officials, community leaders, teachers, and representatives of the Alamo Band of Navajo were are all in attendance. Many speeches were given, most far too long and rambling. A potluck lunch was served as school kids again flocked around the governor for autographs.

While sitting with a few bikers and devouring helpings of barbecued beef and cold fried chicken, I realized that I was beginning to make more personal connections with these cyclists. By this time, most had learned I was a physician, with some reputation around the state and in government circles. Previously, they thought I was an emergency technician. With their new realization, many of them began to respond to me with more attention, more conversation, more overt respect. It was a turnabout I had experienced for more than twenty-five years—namely, that when someone discovers you are a physician, the relationship changes immediately. I again wondered why we don't relate to others from our inherent feelings toward them rather than from a review of their credentials.

We pedaled off from Magdalena in the late afternoon for our last leg of the day, twenty-one miles along the mountains to the town of Socorro. Suddenly, the clear and beautiful cobalt skies filled with thunderstorms left over from the summer's "monsoon" season. Dark, ominous clouds hung over the peaks, and a cold, biting rain began to strike our faces as we traversed the hills east of Magdalena and began our gradual descent into the Rio Grande Valley. Lightning bolts could be seen hitting the valley floor below, only a few miles away.

Despite the gentle downslide, my physical pains began again in earnest. Both legs, feeling like lead, were unable to rotate any faster, even downhill. My buttocks were screaming out with the bruises and abrasions from two long days on my hard, narrow cycling seat. My entire spine felt stiff, and a constant dull headache prevented me from entering a peaceful place with my rhythmic mantra, which I tried to force back into its familiar chant.

Most members of the pack were soon out of sight, pedaling effortlessly into Socorro. For me, the last three miles seemed endless, even though the road was level and headwinds had dissipated. I knew I was within the city limits, but each painful mile seemed to bring me no closer to the final stop, at a park near the railyards. This day's leg had been ninety-six miles; and unlike Monday, I had biked about 90 percent of it. After finally rolling into the park, I bypassed the speeches and opted instead to limp to the designated motel and hide out in a small, stark room.

I had seen no visions, experienced no life-changing bolts of insight, and acquired no sense of peacefulness about my future. Except for the beauty of the land on this second day, the birds and animals I had seen along the route, and the special feelings at Zuni Pueblo, I could grasp nothing of great spiritual significance. I drifted into a brief nap, and let the ibuprofen do its magic on my screaming thighs.

Late that night I came to an important decision about my future course on this trek. I had been envisioning two possible scenarios. One was to ride only the first three days, then return with Fred to Santa Fe after turning over the emergency medical coverage to our paramedic from Clovis. The other, if it were possible, was to ride the full five days to the final destination—at the Texas border just outside the city of Hobbs, in New Mexico's far southern corner—and make this a venture of true epic proportion.

But at that late hour, as another long train rumbled through town, I knew the next day would be the last one for me. The final two days, I was aware, would ironically be the easiest of the five, for the mountains would be behind us and the pedaling—through Roswell, Artesia, Carlsbad, and then Hobbs—would be flat and fast across

New Mexico's portion of the Great Plains. But my knees were already swollen, and ached deeply with a tendinitis that would surely get worse. I had covered the most difficult part of the journey, crossing high mountain passes and the Continental Divide. I had nothing left to prove to myself—except, perhaps, the nagging presence of a clouded stupidity insisting that I could make it all the way.

Yes, Wednesday would be my last day on that bicycle.

DAY 3—WEDNESDAY

We were all up again before dawn, and despite a chill in the air, the day promised to be clear and warmer as we crossed New Mexico's central deserts. This third day would be the longest and most difficult leg— from Socorro across a vast stretch of open desert before finally reaching the Capitán Mountains and Lincoln, some 120 miles away.

But before starting the real journey east, we had an officially scheduled stop that I had been looking forward to for days. Just ten miles south of Socorro lies the tiny village of San Antonio, founded in 1629, which boasts two exceptional historical tidbits. For one, it was the birthplace of hotel magnate Conrad Hilton and site of his first rooms for hire, in a simple little boardinghouse. For another, it is the home of the funkiest, most unusual bar and grill in the Southwest— the famous Owl Cafe.

The Owl—documented birthplace of the official green chile cheeseburger, now an internationally loved dish. The Owl Cafe still makes the best green chile cheeseburgers in the world. It was founded in late 1944 by Frank and Dee Chavez and has been operating contin- ually since then. In 1976 the Chavezes turned it over to their daughter Rowena and her husband, Ray Baca, who run it still. Present-day New Mexicans speak of a time-honored political reality that seldom has been broken: almost no one has ever been elected to high state office without visiting the Owl for a campaign-stop cheeseburger.

But the Owl also has a more serious history, in which locals take even more pride. When Robert Oppenheimer and his cadre of geniuses, hidden up in Los Alamos in World War II, were frantically working on the Manhattan Project to develop the world's first atomic weapon, they chose as the test site for detonation a spot in the isolated desert not far from here. Oppy and his cohorts ate their daily lunch and dinner at the Owl during the final months before the blast, so the story is told, as they worked out their calculations on yellow tablets atop the plain wooden tables.

Over the past twenty years, during countless stops at the Owl Cafe for a green chile cheeseburger, I had often taken a seat in one of the ancient wooden booths and wondered if Oppy once sat right where I was. And could it have been over food at the Owl that he first began to seriously contemplate the universal implications of his up-until-then theoretical work?

To celebrate the governor's ride across the state, Rowena Baca put together a massive traditional breakfast for the group. Breakfast is not typically served at the Owl, but everyone on the staff got up early that morning to help. We entered the cafe's hallowed doors at 7 A.M. and were greeted by tables piled high with scrambled eggs, *papas* (fried potatoes), sausage, bacon, fresh juice, coffee, warm tortillas just off the grill, and of course, large bowls of red and green chile for smothering the eggs. Too much food for everyone—but we devoured it with respect, and with the realization that the day ahead would be very long.

We headed out directly east from San Antonio, taking the gentle road across the wide Rio Grande and the sizable *bosque* on either side of it, where life-sustaining water from the river nourishes broad beltways of tall cottonwood and elm, intrusions of unwelcome salt cedar, and expanses of wetland sanctuaries for migrating birds. The day was warming nicely, and the ride felt smooth and easy.

Over the next few hours we pedaled along the north edge of an area full of history, mystery, and more than its share of misery. Called Jornada del Muerto, or Journey of Death, it is a 200-mile-long, extremely arid valley between the Rio Grande and San Andres Mountains. It was named hundreds of years ago by early conquistadors and missionaries as part of their route on the old Camino Real from Mexico City to the farthest reaches of their empire, in Santa Fe. After leaving the relative comfort of El Paso and Las Cruces, the foreign invaders had to traverse this brutal land, where water sources were a rarity and where if heat and windstorms didn't take a toll on them, the rattlesnakes would. Hence the name of this long-inhospitable valley.

In more modern times, the Jornada del Muerto was a place for the mining of riches, where men often felt it necessary to murder one another for rights to a promising claim. There are countless rumors and old tales of caches of gold and silver hidden up in the foothills, left behind by long-forgotten miners who never made it back to reclaim their fortunes.

This valley of misery has for many decades been off-limits as a military reservation, the White Sands Missile Range. High, formidable chain-link fences surround the bombing-missile test site. Visitors who wander onto the range are usually greeted in short time by soldiers with automatic weapons and attack helicopters.

Only about twenty miles to the south of the road abutting the Jornado del Muerto is where the "most historically significant" event ever to happen in New Mexico took place. At 5:29 A.M. on July 16, 1945, the first nuclear explosion in the history of humankind was detonated from a grotesque-looking experimental bomb called the "thing" or "gadget." A blinding flash of light could be seen from as far as 160 miles away; glass windows shattered in Silver City, some 120 miles to the west; and a deep rumble shook the city of Albuquerque, 100 miles to the north. A crater 400 yards in diameter and eight feet deep was instantly created. The desert sand, exposed to temperatures approaching those of the sun, immediately fused the silicon into a new rock form named trinitite, a starkly beautiful green jadelike substance that can still be found in local rock shops. It was a moment that forever changed the course of human history, and per- haps even the long-term history of earth as a place where diverse life forms can survive.

Ground zero for the blast is called Trinity Site. Although the crater has long since filled in, the spot is marked by a twenty-foot-tall, fairly stark stone obelisk. Twice each year, Trinity Site is open to the public for one day. People flock in by car, RV, and tour bus to have their pictures taken at the monolith, comb the surrounding desert for pieces of trinitite, or silently meditate and pray in remembrance of what happened there.

Our crew of riders stopped for a scheduled water-and-fruit break at Stallion Gate, the entranceway that Oppenheimer and his team passed through to Trinity Site in 1945, and the only access to the site of the public's twice-yearly pilgrimages. A fairly small but official tourist sign stands alongside the road, giving a straightforward history of the thunderous event at a spot just over the southern horizon. As many of the bikers mulled around and talked among themselves, the rest of us stood silently at Stallion's Gate, staring off toward the moment in time that had shaped so much of the world we knew.

We continued east through the desert on a road heading steadily upward toward the San Andres Range far ahead. During the climb, my legs and wind began to give out again. Our next scheduled stop was a ghost town called Bingham, about twenty miles away.

En route to Bingham, something very unusual happened.

I was pedaling along at my traditional plodding pace, with no riders visible either before or behind me, my head lowered toward the roadway, and my mind lost in a hypnotic place, when a flash of movement to the right suddenly caught my eye. I looked toward the high-wire fence of the missile range about twenty feet away. There, running along the fence line was a surreal sight—a large, exotic horned animal about the size of a small elk. Its coat was bright with distinct patterns in white, tan, and black. Its head was primarily white, offset by an almost comical dark mask around the eyes, giving it the appearance of a circus clown. The animal's two black horns were razor-sharp, nearly three feet long, and arching majestically backward from its head in perfect symmetry. It was an oryx, sometimes called a gemstock.

I knew of this animal, although its presence so close to me here in the desolate wilderness of New Mexico immediately struck me as bizarre. Members of the antelope family, these large grazing creatures were imported some twenty-five years ago from Africa and placed in the protective habitat of the missile range. The small initial herd had taken well to the vastness of the desert and, with no natural predators about, had grown into a herd exceeding 1,000 head.

Although it was meant to be fenced in with the others, this solitary oryx had somehow found an opening in the chain links and was running along outside them, very close the road. There was a hint of fear in the animal as it loped along at an easy gallop exactly in concert with my bike. The movement of its legs, rising and falling in rhythmic dance against the earth, was mesmerizing. Each time they completed their cyclic gallop, the air expelled from the animal's massive chest gave forth a guttural sound, like a deep, relaxing sigh of contentment. A moist stain of sweat stood out on its large chest in the bright midday sun.

Our eyes locked often as we moved harmoniously through that place. The fear in its eyes soon gave way to a seemingly profound curiosity.

Except for the oryx and me, everything in my field of vision seemed to blur. As though seen "through a glass darkly," the expanse of desert, its vegetation, and the mountains in the distance became nondistinct; only the sharp colors and unusual silhouette of the oryx seemed in focus. I quickly found myself settling into a matched rhythm with this new companion, in terms of both my pace and my cycle of breathing. I thought of swimming alone with a dolphin in warm southern waters and mystically flying with an eagle over mountaintops. There was a natural peacefulness in the moment.

Before long, I was in an altered state of consciousness. There was no blistering desert heat, no insurmountable hills to climb, no deep burning in my legs. There was no cancer in me or fear of an abbreviated life span. There was only the steady flow of two creatures moving effortlessly through this small piece of the universe.

I felt such comfort and harmony that time passed without me.

The oryx and I ran together for what seemed like miles. Then suddenly, I looked toward the fence line and he was gone. Vanished. Logic begged me to conclude that the animal had found another break in the fence line and had scurried back into the protected confines of the missile range. But how could it have happened so instantaneously? I stopped pedaling at once and looked back across the expanse of open desert to the south. No trees blocked my panoramic view for miles in all directions. I saw no movement or dust trail of an oryx heading back toward its home. I heard no sounds of the gallop of a large animal—just the utter quietness of the desert and a soft breeze rustling the sage and chamisa.

I stayed in that spot many minutes, straddling my bike and straining to catch a glimpse or sound of my companion. As I searched, my mind wandered over matters beyond simple description. Then I pushed on.

Eventually I arrived in Bingham, population twelve. The other bikers had already pedaled in and were enjoying cool drinks and fresh fruit, prepared by a young couple who operated a small store specializing in rocks and gems from the area. As we sat under cooling trees behind their trailer, talk turned to what it was like living in such isolation. Someone in the group asked about the exotic animals now living on the missile range. The young couple's comments about the oryxes gave me a sudden shiver.

Oryxes were considered unpredictable and very dangerous, for they were easily frightened and would charge at the object of fear, their razor-sharp horns lowered in a potentially fatal thrust. Oryxes outside the fence line had been known to charge at cars and spear completely through the metal doors with their horns. To the local state police, they were a nuisance and genuine danger. When one escaped the range, it was typically shot on sight to prevent injury to a traveler.

This description of oryx behavior hardly matched the impression I'd had of my companion a few miles back, for I had never sensed danger. I sat quietly under the shade trees marveling at the disjunction between the frightful reputation of this animal and the peacefulness I had felt moving with it during our time together. Lost in thought, I stared at the desert valley below for a very long time.

The next several miles passed without major events, since my thoughts were no longer on this bike trek but on maintaining the peacefulness I had felt about my critical illness during my time with the oryx. From Bingham we undertook another steady climb, over the Oscura Mountains. Eventually, the range was topped, and I began a gradual, easy ascent into the Tularosa Valley and the village of Carrizozo, our next scheduled rest stop.

Along the way, we crossed a rare geological formation, the *malpais*, or "bad country"—a solidified lava flow from an erupted volcano to the northwest called Little Black Peak. The volcano was active only 1,000 years ago, almost yesterday by geological standards, and had left behind a forty-four-mile-long ribbon of glistening jet-black basalt lava. Because of the fairly recent eruption, the area was nearly devoid of vegetation; in fact, all I could see were the residual caves, tubes, blisters, and bubblelike vesicles. The place felt otherworldly as I pedaled up and down the sinuous road carved out of the lava flow.

By midafternoon, I was sure I had entered another realm. The day reverberated with surreal landscapes and momentous events—yet still one more awaited me, just down the road.

Ten miles outside of Carrizozo I once again found myself at the back of the pack of riders. Though I willed my legs to keep pumping, they were ceasing to function, and with every agonizing turn of the pedals I reconfirmed my decision to finish the journey this day. I had often read of the invisible barrier—the "wall"—that many marathon runners hit in response to the depletion of metabolic foods and fluids, the tortured state that convinces them they can no longer go on. So *this* is what it feels like, I thought. Now I understood why even the most dedicated runners will suddenly quit, despite all their determination, compulsiveness, and months of training. This was just too painful to endure.

I finally reached the Carrizozo park, where hamburgers and fresh fruit waited. I could not face the food, but forced down enough liquid to alleviate some of the pain. There was now no doubt in my mind: not only would this be my last day on the trek, but this spot right here, under the ramada in Carrizozo, would be where I put my bike away for the final time. I could no longer keep up the charade.

I felt a certain peacefulness in the surrender. I harbored not a sense of failure, but rather a harmony that had come with the quest—and the chance meeting with the oryx. I told Fred of my decision, and he understood immediately.

After throwing my bike in the back of our emergency van, I rode for the rest of the thirty miles to Lincoln with Fred, assisting him in treating the growing number of riders experiencing muscle cramps, hyperthermia, and dizziness. One by one, more of them opted to ride in the chase van for the rest of the day. Others—driven by unspoken internal needs—struggled on, even though I saw signs of confusion and profuse sweating that indicated progressive hyperthermia.

We rested briefly in tiny Capitán, an enchanting mountain community that in May of 1950, when a raging forest fire destroyed thousands of acres of pine trees to the north, gave the world a frightened, badly burned black bear cub that eventually was named Smokey Bear; he lived out his life in the National Zoo in Washington, DC, as the symbol of the country's forest-fire prevention program. The last ten miles were through high mountain passes into historic Lincoln, a place that has successfully defied time. This was the center of the Lincoln County range wars, which brought to public attention the larger-than-life personas of William "Billy the Kid" Bonney, Sheriff Pat Garrett, and the rest.

Sitting on the steps of the Lincoln County Courthouse, from which Billy the Kid escaped the day before his scheduled hanging, I exchanged goodbyes and remembrances with the support crew and my fellow riders. Many of the interactions were warm, deserving of the closeness we had experienced together during our personal struggles over the previous three days. I spent time in private with the governor, assuring him of the emergency response we had arranged for the last two days of the trip. We also spoke honestly about physical challenges, and the beauty of the places we had been to.

Come early evening, Fred and I were off in the van, heading back to Santa Fe. Despite my physical exhaustion, I drove most of the way as Fred rested from the understandable mental fatigue that had come from driving at ten miles an hour for the better part of three days. Neither of us felt like talking. I was thankful for the solitude and the time to reflect on the long stretches of desolate roads behind us. I thought deeply about the separate reality I had felt with the oryx. I remembered the loneliness and pain of the bike trek as well as the previous four years of my life. And I again felt the solitudinous essence of my days.

Many other aspects of the trip would be considered in the future. But at the moment, all I could contemplate was the throbbing pain in my legs and back, a numbing headache, my sunburned skin, and my compelling need to be home again.

EPILOGUE

Major leaps in the core of our spirit are seldom obvious. We go on from day to day, making the same assumptions and reacting with habitual impulses despite the fact that something important has happened within us. Visions, too, are subtle—no burning bushes or voices from the clouds of lore and legend. New insights have to be shaped by time before becoming part of the psyche.

I came back from the long bike journey with more than swollen knees and sunburned skin. It took time and reflection to feel the changes intensely, but I had no doubt of their existence. For one thing, I decided to undergo eight weeks of radiation therapy to my neck—a last-ditch effort to stem the progress of my malignancy. Despite the low odds of success and inevitably nasty side effects, I had felt such an intensity of life during the three days of biking that any chance to stave off mortality was worth the effort.

For another, I rediscovered pride in my physical essence, however withered it was by age, malignancy, and frequent surgeries. I appreciated my capacity to face a major health challenge and still surmount the endless hills on each new horizon.

But most importantly, it was again emblazoned upon my spirit that beauty and connectedness permeate the earth, sky, clouds, and all things. There is a balance to the fitting together of our universe, as is sung in my favorite Navajo healing chant:

> All is beautiful before me
> behind me
> below me
> above me.
> All is beautiful all around me.

I've had frequent dreams of running with the oryx. I see the shimmering sweat on his muscular chest and hear the guttural sound of his exhalations as he moves along in a smooth gallop. I feel safe with him. Although the oryx, like my cancer, is said to be bizarre and rare and deadly, he evokes no fear or sense of danger. To the contrary, he inspires a harmony, a lasting peacefulness.

I am now more at peace with the fatal illness within, no matter what course it may take as time passes. Although it will undoubtedly be the final cause of my death and transition to some other reality, my malignancy has also been an intense source of energy that has allowed me to visit special places of the soul.

Like the oryx, it has been a strange and powerful visitor in my life, with a special message that comes in times of solitude and silence.

Forced Silence

MY FORCED SILENCE CAME ON SUDDENLY one morning. Awakening from an intense dream, I headed for the bathroom; then as the psychotic family cat scurried by my foot, I opened my mouth to voice her name in greeting. Nothing came out, however, except a whisper of windy exhalation. No noticeable sound, no distinguishable words. Just a rush of silence.

Damn, I thought. That's strange.

But it was not strange. I should have sensed it coming, since I was in the midst of a six-week course of radiation to my throat for this recurrent malignancy. The silence had been foretold by the doctor and nurse at the cancer treatment center. It had been right there in handwritten script on the patient consent form I had signed before treatments began: "Persistent sore throat, difficulty swallowing, changes in normal voice patterns."

Still, its suddenness and completeness took me by surprise. And for the next five weeks, contending with forced silence was a constant reality.

Over four years of dealing with the highs and lows of this illness, a score of numbing reactions, complications, cosmetic disruptions, and transient disabilities had been visiting me like unwanted, bad houseguests. The unpleasant visitors, while intense at the time, were on hindsight less painful and emotionally present.

Even so, I remembered them all. The long recuperation from skull-base surgery in Texas, when I was burdened with persistent draining fistulas, facial paralysis, and the grotesque appearance that comes with a radical neck procedure. The four-month loss of taste following my first course of radiation, which took away one of the great joys of my life—savoring the delectable essence of food and wine. And the constant, unhealing skin burns on my neck from the insult of radiation on those dermal cells that would otherwise give birth to new, healthy tissue.

But this silence felt different. Although it quickly evolved into a psychological pain, it coincidentally also became a kind teacher that opened up poignant matters of the spirit.

The first, most memorable consequence I felt occurred while trying to order food. Whether it was coffee and a doughnut in the morning or a Big Mac around noon, I quickly found that walking up to the counter to place an order became a humiliating, frustrating experience. The young salesperson would stare at me with a look of frightened concern as I tried to articulate loudly enough to be understood. Typically, two or three attempts at labored words, reading lips, pointing to coffee urns, and other body language were needed to get across the message.

I became so self-conscious of the fragility of simple communication that I began to shy away from public interactions where I might be forced to talk. Rather than ordering meals at fast-food places, I survived on tasteless, generic ham sandwiches from the refrigerated section of a convenience store. I used automatic teller machines instead of going face-to-face with bank clerks. I'd let the telephone ring on and on, even when people knew I was at home, fearing the embarrassment of trying to say hello.

The forced silence, which intensified as the weeks of radiation continued, caused me to turn inside myself, forsaking the human contact that fills much of our days. I withdrew more and more, refusing to go out to dinner with my wife or socialize with friends. Like a telescope used in reverse, the silence of my voice reflected inwardly to my deepest parts, where I found a safer place. There I could communicate with ease, sing with wonderful gusto, and reweave old Irish tales I had read in books. There I was not disabled or encumbered.

Yet this forced withdrawal into self came at a bad time. As other physical symptoms of the radiation appeared—pain, constant throaty secretions, weight loss—my heaviness of spirit intensified. This was the fourth year of the malignant madness, compounded with what seemed like recurrence after recurrence despite the full array of both Western and alternative healing practices I had embraced. Although going inside to a safe port allayed my fears of communicating, it was not at all helpful in maintaining a healing optimism or accepting good energy from those who cared. On the contrary, it brought me to a place that was private and dark, where I felt utterly alone.

So I tried consciously to turn the silence around, to make it an ally rather than a drain. Over time, that conscious effort seemed to work, becoming a ticket to more important matters of spirit.

At first, I focused on the cloistered monks of untold centuries who made vows of silence to their god as reflections of piety and devotion. Their voices were restricted to chants, and then only on rare occasions. The images of these hooded monks often gave me a measure of strength. That strength came not from their affiliation with a particular religious sect, but from the dignity of discipline for a cause, as exhibited through their vows.

I focused, too, on images of isolated Buddhist monasteries high in the Himalayas, where devotees of contemplative practices spend their entire lives in silence and meditation—all intended to reach a point of harmony and oneness with the universe as they envision it. In addition, I thought of young Native American men on their vision quests, isolating themselves for weeks in shallow caves deep in the mountains, never speaking so as not to interrupt the spirit messages from the earth, which would direct them to future paths.

Centering on these images while turning off connections with the outside world stimulated an experience of the kindness of the universe in a way that the latest TV episode of *Seinfeld* never could. Much time was spent staring at clouds as they changed ever so slowly, watching color burst forth in evening sunsets, listening to the sounds of old forgotten music pulled from dusty cartons to bring back flashes of happiness. Like a blinded person who develops hyperacute hearing, taste, and touch, I found that my forced silence opened corridors of perception and mindfulness that helped me face my illness and fear of imminent mortality.

My voice eventually began to return, slowly. Every so often between the forced whispers, a loud sound would suddenly, unpredictably, burst forth. The rare intelligible words gradually became sentences, then entire thoughts. I could stand at a counter and order a pizza to go. I could answer the phone. I could express a feeling of affection for someone close.

Like a person who is reunited with a long-lost friend and stays up all night sharing missed experiences, I then entered a brief hyperactive phase of talking too much. At work meetings, I would verbally interrupt to make a point, however mundane. I babbled on and on with fairly uninteresting observations that no one really wanted to hear. I sang out loud to music on the car radio while driving home in the evening.

Ultimately, I returned to my more recognizable self—someone who is relatively taciturn, except when there is a message to convey. My frenzy of verbal communication, although intense, was short-lived.

What remained were memories of the places I had frequented in my spirit and psyche during that time of forced silence. To this day, I remember the fears and isolation and withdrawal into the dark side, which are now part of dreams. But more importantly, I remember the places of strength and harmony I visited. Embedded within me, they help carry me through the frightening uncertainties of future days.

The Caregivers

I AM DYING OF CANCER. Now in my early fifties, I should be in the prime of my life. Instead, the last five years have been filled with fluctuations between hope and resignation, remissions countered with unexpected relapses, and seemingly successful interventions such as surgery and radiation that have left their marks of lingering disability and compromise. In short, I have been thrust into the frightening role of a patient with a critical medical condition.

I've spent days and nights looking back on my career, marveling at the incredible work we physicians do. What brings us to this unique and powerful position? What are the seminal events that have shaped my own abilities as a healer? These questions frequently return me to a night nearly thirty years ago, which gives me a measure of strength to face the lonely moments of terror and sadness.

It was the summer of 1969 in oppressively hot and humid Philadelphia, and I was beginning my third year in medical school at the University of Pennsylvania. I had just finished up the two long years of required basic sciences—anatomy, physiology, pharmacology, and a score of other "ologies" that form the core of medical education. My fellow students and I were finally let loose in the hospital environment to make that critical transition from book learning to dealing with actual patients and complex medical problems that could never be captured in textbooks.

We had no experience with patient care, but certainly knew how to dress for the part. We marched with pride around the hospital in our brand-new white coats, pockets overflowing with stethoscopes, reflex hammers, notebooks, and study guides outlining appropriate history and assessment techniques. Our shortened uniforms identified our lowly status to all hospital staff, easily separating our importance from that of the interns, residents, and other "real" doctors.

My first clinical rotation that summer was in obstetrics-gynecology. Some wise professor must have figured out that as completely naive student doctors, we would do less harm here than in other rotations—largely because 90 percent of babies born over the course of human existence have come screaming into the world on their own initiative, without the intervention of a doctor to complicate matters.

Most births seemed to occur in the early morning hours. On this particular night at 2:00 A.M., I was part of a team that included an attending professor, two or three OB-GYN resident physicians, an intern or two, a fourth-year medical student on elective, and—at the bottom of the pecking order—me, shuffling behind in my little white coat. This small army of white coats would rush around the hospital like a school of fish, with the attending physician throwing out difficult questions on patient care, most of which were directed at me. I was in a constant state of insecurity and awkwardness as I watched this hierarchy of practitioners flow effortlessly from evaluating patients to making quick, critical decisions. I practiced my interviewing techniques with an authoritative tone, but inherently knew the charade was rarely believed.

During this late shift, we were evaluating twenty-four-year-old Leana, a rather large African American woman from the poorest neighborhood in West Philly. She was about to give birth to her fourth child. Her other labors had been fairly smooth, but this one would be different. The fetus was horizontal in the uterus, rather than head down. Leana was in her eighth hour of intense labor, and the infant was not about to turn starboard. Since the fetus's vital signs were beginning to deteriorate, the various physicians, residents, and interns began scurrying about in all directions to prepare for a cesarean section. At that point, the chief OB resident called out to me, "You stay with the patient and keep on top of things."

Keep on top of things? Was he out of his mind? The closest I'd ever been to a real delivery was while watching my family dog give birth to a litter of six.

I stood by the bedside and feebly tried to reassure this sizable patient who was screeching obscenities and threatening to kill the first man who came into her field of vision. Suddenly, in a moment of agony, she blindly reached out and grabbed my hand with enough pressure, I was sure, to compromise my blood supply. I don't think she knew she had latched onto me, or that I represented anything more to her than a stationary object in her world of confusion and pain. I instinctively tried to pull away from her, for it seemed some official barrier had been breeched.

Then something important happened. The intense hand grip seemed to quiet the chaos of her hurt and fear. As I gradually relaxed into this deeply personal connection, I found myself softly intoning words of comfort and support. Her breathing slowed, and the screams abated. My identity as a budding doctor versed in book knowledge evaporated in the midst of giving the only things I could offer—my concern and the reassurance of a human presence.

We sat in silence, holding hands for what seemed like an eternity, until the operating room crew came to take her away. A healthy nine-pound baby was delivered by cesarean section shortly thereafter. As I stood at her bedside with our team of physicians during morning rounds the next few days, neither she nor I ever acknowledged what had happened between us.

Up to that point, I had been someone merely learned in the sciences, compulsive enough to do well in college courses and on entrance exams. Becoming a doctor seemed like a natural progression for me, and it had all been quite easy until then. But the profound moment of connection with a patient in pain at 2 A.M. on a stifling hot summer night—together with the feeling that this helped dissipate her misery—was one of those critical turning points that can be neither planned nor repeated. It converted me from a scientist to a caregiver.

This transformation reverberated throughout my career. I finished the last two furious years of medical school and then went on to internship, where sleep was an unknown luxury and the mundane chores in patient care were expected requirements. After that, it resounded continually as I spent over eight years living and working in isolated reservation settings. It even sustained me through the long months of providing rural primary care and the subsequent seventeen years of intense practice as an emergency physician at a chaotically busy hospital.

Yes, I was meant to be a caregiver. Certainly, there have been financial rewards and trappings of prestige and power that come with being a physician in our culture. But those "perks" have always paled in comparison to the heady feeling of being called upon to help someone in need.

At times it has felt more like a curse. Incalculable interludes of sleep deprivation have strained my tolerance, as well as my family's. Numerous legitimate frustrations have accompanied the realization that 80 percent of what brings patients to doctors is caused by the disharmony of spirit and body rather than microbes and infective agents. Working with disenfranchised groups like Native Americans and Latinos, I have come face-to-face with the depression and misery that modern society has forced on the human spirit; patients are frequently angry, violent, and hateful toward those trying to provide care. Moreover, I've been concerned with unresolvable problems such as unequal access to all levels of treatment, restrictive policies of managed care, and the often cold and impersonal facade of Western medicine. Throughout these past twenty-seven years, my joy in being a caregiver has been severely tested.

Still, I am grateful for having served in that special position all this time! I sense a similar gratitude among many of those I have been honored to work with: nurses, techs, complementary healers, and the EMTs providing field care. Although we all get an adrenalin rush from the flashing lights and busy emergency rooms, we also experience a compelling impulse to help others—often despite great discomfort—when the call comes in or the beeper goes off.

For me, now is a time of remembrance rather than long-range planning. Personally contending with a bizarre malignancy has meant multiple surgeries and radiation treatments, with periods of some stability inevitably followed by recurrences. It has now become obvious that the cancer has turned quite nasty again and will eventually prevail. It appears quite certain that the time has come for me to put aside matters of being a physician and move toward another transition, whatever that may entail.

As I move on to devote more time to family and other personal concerns, I often become locked in reverie and memories. That hot summer night with Leana three decades ago radiates in all its vividness. The days ahead will be spent collecting such moments and closing the sacred loops. I will write, take long mountain walks, listen to loud, loud music—and remember how blessed I am for having had the opportunity to be a caregiver.

Closing Prayer

Today is a very good day to die.
Every living thing is in harmony with me.
Every voice sings a chorus within me.
All beauty has come to rest in my eyes.
All bad thoughts have departed from me.
Today is a very good day to die.
My land is peaceful around me.
My fields have been turned for the last time.
My house is filled with laughter.
My children have come home.
Yes, today is a very good day to die.

—NANCY WOOD

Afterword

Tim Fleming was a quiet man. Far more resonant than the timbre of his voice were the triumphs of his too-short life.

Many people knew Tim as a doctor to the Indians. His first work after medical training was in the canyon country of Arizona, where he remains the healer who set the standard by which all his successors were measured by members of the Hualapai and Havasupai tribes, even twenty-five years after he left.

Many knew Tim as an emergency-room physician. For seventeen years he dealt with the constant flow of crisis at northern New Mexico's largest hospital. Again he excelled—gaining board certification, teaching university students, becoming director of the state's Emergency Medical Services Bureau.

A few fortunate people knew Tim as a member of their family— as son, brother, husband, father, uncle, cousin.

But I . . . I knew Tim as a writer.

Our first meeting was auspicious. As editor of the struggling, fledgling *Santa Fe Reporter* in New Mexico's capital city, I presided over an enterprise that threatened with each week's issue to come unstuck. Most salaries were about $140 a week, our equipment was antiquated, and paying the bills was a monthly juggling act. But we kept coming out.

Tuesday was deadline day, and it lasted until 4 o'clock Wednesday morning, the final moment we could get the pages to the printer in time. One Tuesday evening in 1975, a staff member brought a friend in with her for the late-night push. He was a lanky fellow named Tim Fleming, and he said that although he was a doc, he had this thing about newspapers. If he stayed out of our way, could he watch for a while?

He slipped into the background, observing all dozen of us rushing through our tasks. Then shortly before midnight, disaster struck. Our lone typesetter got sick. Though others could run the machine, everybody had urgent work to do. For the first time ever, it seemed we might miss our deadline.

"Your machine looks like a fairly basic word processor, and I'm a fairly decent typist," a soft voice said. "If you set it up for me, I might be able to lend a hand." Then for the next four hours, Tim Fleming brought the paper home.

We offered repeatedly to spell him; but he said no, he was holding up fine. At some point I realized that his modest "helping hand" had become a personal challenge and a thrill for Tim. I also realized that here was a remarkable man.

Just how remarkable I continued to learn. A few weeks later he casually dropped off a feature-length manuscript, about Old Duke, an aged medicine man he met as an Indian Health Service doctor with the Hualapai Nation in Arizona. "I do a little writing on the side," he said. His story was rich, colorful, and mysterious. We displayed it prominently.

Early in 1978 the *Reporter's* one sports writer gave notice. Soon Tim was in my office, proposing something in his soft voice. "This is nuts, Tim," I replied. "You can't take a break from medicine and work for us full-time. You're a doctor! You actually make money. Do you know what we pay?"

"Of course I do," he said. "And I know what I'm doing."

For the next eight months, Tim was our sports department.

His very first story was about his favorite subject: the University of New Mexico Lobos men's basketball team. The *Reporter* had a decidedly local emphasis, in sports as well as the rest of the paper. But Tim figured, rightly, that the big-time Lobos had thousands of Santa Fe fans.

In Tim's one bright shining season, UNM had perhaps its most flamboyant team ever, averaging more than 100 points a game for weeks and ranking as high as No. 4 nationally. And Tim ate it up. He got full press credentials, and covered most home games courtside. He sat at a long table among the visiting pros from *Sports Illustrated,* the *Denver Post* and NBC Sports, and gave them insider tips. Nowhere was he more happy than in the deafening roar of the Pit. And when the Lobos choked in the NCAA tournament, he was inconsolable.

Well, for a day or two anyway. Tim actually was so busy doing everything required of a one-man sports department he had no time to mope. In each issue he was responsible for two or three lengthy articles and several local briefs. It was a lot of work for a rookie. But not enough for Tim.

After just a few weeks he started writing a personal column as well, which he called "One on One." His subjects ranged from Muhammad Ali to frisbees to Little League. And though we had a staff photographer, Tim wanted to take his own pictures. He also did his own layouts and headlines.

He wasn't polished at the start. But he was as quick a study as I had ever taught. He kept on getting better. So did his section. He appreciated almost everything in the wide world of sports, and wrote about most of it. Billiards, prep football, Santa Fe Downs, marathoners, gliders, girls' softball. One issue featured Pete Rose—and miniature golf.

The day came when Tim told me, in his soft voice, that "he'd enjoyed as much of this as he could stand." The news saddened but did not surprise me. For Tim was a caregiver.

He joined the emergency-room staff at Santa Fe's only hospital, St. Vincent. Soon he was sending stories again to the *Reporter:* about Christmas in the emergency room, about removing organs from dying crash victims to give new life to other patients. His emergency-room account of the horrendous 1980 New Mexico prison riot, in which thirty-three inmates died, won the state's top award for medical writing. His "The Real ER" opened some star-struck eyes: "It isn't TV or the movies."

In 1988 I sold the *Reporter.* Tim and I kept in touch, going to Lobo games, meeting at parties, having lunch. Then at lunch one day in 1993, I learned why his voice was soft. Twenty-six years earlier he had lost a vocal cord to cancer. For all the intervening years he had thought he was cured. But now the malignancy had returned, aggressively. He was in for a fight. But medicine had come a long way since the 1960s.

Next came surgery, then radiation, then more surgery, more radiation, more surgery. Tim was fighting valiantly but losing ground. When we met he spoke of the inexorable, the inevitable. But there was a job he wanted to tackle first.

He set a typewritten manuscript on the table. "Let me know what you think of this," he said. I read it at once and called him. "It's terrific, Tim. It's got to be published!"

But he was racing against time, against death. "Maybe a month and a half," Tim estimated his prognosis. "That's not long enough to get a book out," I had to tell him. "Well, let's get started on it," he replied. "My dream is to hold my book in my hands. But if I don't get to do that, just knowing it's in the pipeline will mean a lot. We'll see."

That was in October 1998. To speed the process, Tim asked me to edit his collection, just as I had given a last read to his work at the *Reporter* twenty years earlier. But even after my input, Tim had the final say. I worked as quickly as possible, zipped my changes to Tim, and he decided which to keep and which to override. It was essential that his ultimate statement speak in the sound of *his* soft voice.

November slid into December, 1998 into 1999. We stayed in almost constant touch, and late into the nights Tim sat at his keyboard, punching in the finished version. I feared for his stamina. Yet he seemed to grow stronger, not weaker. "He's determined to see this through," a friend explained.

I was not surprised. Once again Tim had taken on an astonishing challenge. Again he refused to fail the test. Bonding with his words at my own keyboard, I marveled at what he had crafted. Through pain and fear and ebbing strength, he had erected three pillars on which to place his testament. "Indian Ways" blended an almost mystical comprehension of Native American worlds with the personal development of a young physician. "The Seduction of Trauma" pulsed with adrenaline—and compassion. "Gathering Shadows" stared unblinkingly into the eyes of his impending death.

I pictured Tim pulling his memories and reflections together, knowing that the time was short, the end near. I watched him pause for the latest surgery, and the long recuperation. I saw his hopes rise, only to fall once more. Then back he went to his desk. It was hard to believe.

And now, in this last great push, he wanted the work to be *good.* Flogging his depleted body on, he made arrangements with a book publisher, a designer, photographers, a poet, other authors. He conferred with me on fine points of the writer's craft, and wrestled with rewrites after we talked. Yes, Tim was determined to see this thing through.

March arrived, and with it *A Rendezvous With Clouds.* Tim got his wish: to hold his book in his hands, to inscribe copies to his wife, to his three children, to the people dearest in his life. But he also got much more than that.

He lived to see early reviews of *A Rendezvous With Clouds.* One said: "Other physicians have written about facing life-threatening illnesses, but few have had such a rich journey to that point in their lives." Another added: "Not only are his stories spellbinding in their insight, humanity and humility, the writing itself demonstrates how personal nonfiction can rise to the level of literature."

He lived to preside happily over a major book-signing event at a fine resort in Santa Fe. Hundreds of friends and acquaintances and strangers came, to buy hundreds of his books, in which he scribbled the perfect personal touch.

He lived to see most of his book's initial print run, from the small Chamisa Press in Santa Fe, sell out. And he lived long enough to see the University of New Mexico Press eagerly take on "A Rendezvous With Clouds" for this edition. And then, perhaps, Tim was satisfied that the job was done.

Tim died on April 20, 1999, at the age of fifty-four. At his memorial service, many people spoke: family members, poker buddies, doctors, neighbors, lawyers, Santa Fe's fire chief, tribal officials and other Indians, ambulance drivers and friends. All brought their own special memories. I spoke too. I remembered Tim as a writer—and a remarkable man.

—Richard McCord
June 1999

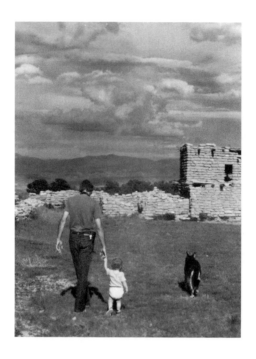

TIM FLEMING, MD (1945–1999), was a board-certified emergency medicine physician who lived north of Santa Fe, New Mexico, with his wife and two children. In addition to his long career as a practitioner with Indian Health Service and as an emergency physician, he served as a health-care administrator as well as a consultant to state, local, and national organizations and Indian tribes. The author of numerous essays published in local and national publications, he was an assistant professor of emergency medicine at the University of New Mexico at the time of his death.

The Timothy T. Fleming, MD Professorship in Emergency Medicine

University of New Mexico School of Medicine

In academia, an endowed professorship is the highest honor bestowed upon an individual. The Timothy T. Fleming, MD Professorship in Emergency Medicine memorializes a husband, father, author, and physician who succeeded in not only saving the lives of individuals but also in improving the health and well-being of entire communities. His passion for health care and his desire to make a difference in people's lives is reflected and honored in this professorship.

The UNM School of Medicine created the Fleming Professorship to educate aspiring physicians, EMTs, and nurses both on progressive methods for the alleviation of suffering and in life-saving stabilizing care prior to hospitalization. Another component will be training in disaster medicine and the delivery of health care when mass casualties occur.

If you would like to make a donation to support this endowed professorship, please mail your tax deductible gift to:

Timothy T. Fleming MD Professorship
UNM Foundation
Two Woodward Center
700 Lomas Blvd. NE, Suite 203
Albuquerque, New Mexico 87131-3196